Geriatric Anesthesia

Editor

SHAMSUDDIN AKHTAR

ANESTHESIOLOGY CLINICS

www.anesthesiology.theclinics.com

Consulting Editor
LEE A. FLEISHER

September 2023 • Volume 41 • Number 3

ELSEVIER

1600 John F. Kennedy Boulevard • Suite 1800 • Philadelphia, Pennsylvania, 19103-2899

http://www.theclinics.com

ANESTHESIOLOGY CLINICS Volume 41, Number 3
September 2023 ISSN 1932-2275, ISBN-13: 978-0-443-18179-5

Editor: Joanna Gascoine
Developmental Editor: Anita Chamoli

Anesthesiology Clinics (ISSN 1932-2275) is published quarterly by Elsevier Inc., 360 Park Avenue South, New York, NY 10010-1710. Months of issue are March, June, September, and December. Periodicals postage paid at New York, NY and at additional mailing offices. Subscription prices are $100.00 per year (US student/resident), $386.00 per year (US individuals), $478.00 per year (Canadian individuals), $740.00 per year (US institutions), $936.00 per year (Canadian institutions), $100.00 per year (Canadian student/resident), $513.00 per year (foreign student/resident), $498.00 per year (foreign individuals), and $936.00 per year (foreign institutions). To receive student and resident rate, orders must be accompanied by name of affiliated institution, date of term, and the *signature* of program/residency coordinator on institutions letterhead. Orders will be billed at individual rate until proof of status is received. Foreign air speed delivery is included in all *Clinics'* subscription prices. All prices are subject to change without notice. POSTMASTER: Send address changes to *Anesthesiology Clinics,* Elsevier Health Sciences Division, Subscription Customer Service, 3251 Riverport Lane, Maryland Heights, MO 63043. Customer Service (orders, claims, online, change of address): Elsevier Health Sciences Division, Subscription Customer Service, 3251 Riverport Lane, Maryland Heights, MO 63043. **Tel:1-800-654-2452 (U.S. and Canada); 314-447-8871 (outside U.S. and Canada). Fax: 314-447-8029. E-mail: journalscustomerservice-usa@elsevier.com (for print support); journalsonlinesupport-usa@elsevier.com (for online support).**

Reprints. For copies of 100 or more of articles in this publication, please contact the Commercial Reprints Department, Elsevier Inc., 360 Park Avenue South, New York, NY 10010-1710. Tel.: 212-633-3874; Fax: 212-633-3820; E-mail: reprints@elsevier.com.

Anesthesiology Clinics, is also published in Spanish by McGraw-Hill Inter-americana Editores S. A., P.O. Box 5-237, 06500 Mexico D. F., Mexico.

Anesthesiology Clinics, is covered in *MEDLINE/PubMed (Index Medicus), Current Contents/Clinical Medicine, Excerpta Medica, ISI/BIOMED,* and *Chemical Abstracts.*

Contributors

CONSULTING EDITOR

LEE A. FLEISHER, MD
Emeritus Professor and Former Chair of Anesthesiology and Critical Care, Perelman School of Medicine, University of Pennsylvania, Philadelphia, Pennsylvania, USA

EDITOR

SHAMSUDDIN AKHTAR, MD, FASA
Professor, Department of Anesthesiology and Pharmacology, Fellowship Director, Critical Care Anesthesiology, Yale School of Medicine, New Haven, Connecticut, USA

AUTHORS

ANTHONY RAY ABSALOM, MBChB, FRCA, MD (UCT)
Professor, Department of Anesthesiology, University of Groningen, University Medical Center Groningen, Groningen, the Netherlands

AMIT BARDIA, MBBS, MPH
Department of Anesthesiology, Critical Care and Pain Medicine, Massachusetts General Hospital, Boston, Massachusetts, USA

MAREK BRZEZINSKI, MD, PhD
Department of Anesthesia and Perioperative Care, University of California, San Francisco VA Medical Center, San Francisco, California, USA

ZYAD J. CARR, MD
Department of Anesthesiology, Yale School of Medicine, New Haven, Connecticut, USA

ELISABETTA CERUTTI, MD
Head, Anestesia e Rianimazione dei Trapianti e Chirurgia Maggiore, Azienda Ospedaliero Universitaria delle Marche, Azienda Ospedaliero Universitaria "Ospedali Riuniti," Ancona, Italy

ROBERT M. CHOW, MD
Department of Anesthesiology, Yale School of Medicine, New Haven, Connecticut, USA

ADRIENNE L. CLARK, MD
Department of Anesthesia and Perioperative Care, University of California, San Francisco, San Francisco, California, USA

ETTIENNE COETZEE, MBChB, MMed, FCA (SA)
Doctor, Department of Anaesthesia and Perioperative Medicine, Groote Schuur Hospital, Cape Town, Republic of South Africa

ROBERT P. DAVIS, MD
Division of Cardiac Surgery, Department of Surgery, Yale School of Medicine, New Haven, Connecticut, USA

HANS D. DE BOER, MD, PhD
Senior Consultant, Department of Anesthesia, Pain Medicine and Procedural Sedation and Analgesia Martini General Hospital Groningen, Van Swietenplein, Groningen, the Netherlands

ANDREA DE GASPERI, MD
Formerly Chair, Anestesia Rianimazione 2 ASST GOM Niguarda, Milan, Italy

STACIE G. DEINER, MD
Professor of Anesthesiology and LeRoy Garth Vice Chair for Research, Department of Anesthesiology, Dartmouth Hitchcock Medical Center, Lebanon, NH, USA

ANDRE F. GOSLING, MD
Department of Anesthesiology and Perioperative Medicine, The University of Alabama at Birmingham, Birmingham, Alabama, USA

WILLIAM K. HART, MD
Assistant Professor, Department of Anesthesiology, University of Vermont Larner College of Medicine, Burlington, VT, USA

ERIN ISAZA, BS
University of California, San Francisco School of Medicine, San Francisco, California, USA

JOHN C. KLICK, MD, FCCP, FASE, FCCM
Associate Professor, Department of Anesthesiology, University of Vermont Larner College of Medicine, Burlington, VT, USA

JASLEEN KUKREJA, MD, MPH
Division of Cardiothoracic Surgery, Department of Surgery, University of California, San Francisco, California, USA

OLLE LJUNGQVIST, MD, PhD
Senior Professor, Department of Surgery, School of Medical Sciences, Örebro University, Örebro, Sweden

ELIZABETH MAHANNA-GABRIELLI, MD
Associate Professor, Department of Anesthesiology, Perioperative Medicine and Pain Management, University of Miami Miller School of Medicine, Miami, Florida, USA

BRITTANY J. MCDOWELL, MD
Department of Anesthesiology, Intermountain Medical Center, Murray, Utah, USA

DOMAGOJ MLADINOV, MD, PhD
Department of Anesthesiology, Perioperative and Pain Medicine, Brigham and Women's Hospital, Boston, Massachusetts, USA

JESSICA NG, MD
Department of Anesthesiology, Yale School of Medicine, New Haven, Connecticut, USA

BHOUMESH PATEL, MD
Division of Cardiac Anesthesiology, Department of Anesthesiology, Yale School of Medicine, New Haven, Connecticut, USA

LAURA PETRÒ, MD
Staff Anesthesiologist, ANRI1–Emergency and Intensive Care, ASST Ospedale Giovanni XXIII, ASST Papa Giovanni XXII, Bergamo, Italy

KANISHKA RAJPUT, MD, FASA
Assistant Professor, Department of Anesthesiology, Yale School of Medicine, New Haven, Connecticut, USA

SIAVOSH SAATEE, MD
Department of Anesthesiology, Feinberg School of Medicine, Chicago, Illinois, USA

MANI RATNESH S. SANDHU, MD
Department of Neurosurgery, University of Iowa Hospitals and Clinics, Iowa City, Iowa, USA

KATIE J. SCHENNING, MD, MPH, MCR
Associate Professor of Anesthesiology and Perioperative Medicine, Assistant Medical Director, Preoperative Medicine Clinic, Department of Anesthesiology and Perioperative Medicine, Oregon Health & Science University, Portland, Oregon, USA

SAUL SILLER, MD
Department of Anesthesiology, Yale School of Medicine, New Haven, Connecticut, USA

MAYANKA TICKOO, MD, MS
Division of Pulmonary Medicine, Department of Medicine, Critical Care and Sleep Medicine, Tufts Medical Center, Boston, Massachusetts, USA

MITCHELL H. TSAI, MD, MMM, FASA, FAACD
Professor, Departments of Anesthesiology, Orthopaedics and Rehabilitation (by courtesy), and Surgery (by courtesy), University of Vermont Larner College of Medicine, Burlington, Vermont, USA

NICHOLAS ZWOLINSKI, MD
Department of Anesthesiology, Yale School of Medicine, New Haven, Connecticut, USA

Contents

With a rapidly aging population and increasing global surgical volumes, managing the elevated risk of perioperative pulmonary complications has become an expanding focus for quality improvement in health care. In this narrative review, we will analyze the evidence-based literature to provide high-quality and actionable management strategies to better detect, stratify risk, optimize, and manage perioperative pulmonary complications in geriatric populations.

Anesthesiologists are increasingly required to care for frail elderly patients. A detailed knowledge of the influence of age on the pharmacokinetics and dynamics of the anesthetic drugs is essential for optimal safety and care. For most of the anesthetic drugs, the elderly need lower doses to achieve the same plasma concentrations, and at any given plasma and effect-site concentration, they will have more profound clinical effects than younger patients. Caution is required, with close monitoring of clinical effects and active titration of dose administration to achieve the desired level of effect, ideally following the "start low, go slow" principle.

A strong association between frailty and in-hospital delirium in nonsurgical patients has been shown. Physical and cognitive frailties have been associated with decline and dysfunction in the frontal cognitive domains. Risk factors for frailty are similar to risk factors for postoperative delirium (POD). Frailty can be screened and diagnosed by various tools and instruments. Different anesthetic techniques have been studied to decrease the incidence of POD. However, no anesthetic technique has been conclusively proven to decrease the risk of POD. Patients with dementia develop delirium more often, and delirium is associated with accelerated cognitive decline.

challenges that data scientists face when focusing on geriatric perioperative research.

Enhanced recovery after surgery (ERAS) is a new way of working where evidence-based care elements are assembled to form a care pathway involving the patient's entire journey through surgery. Many elements included in ERAS have stress-reducing effects on the body or helps avoid side effects associated with alternative treatment options. This leads to less overall stress from the injury caused by the operation and helps facilitate recovery. In old, frail patients with concomitant diseases and less physical reserves, this may help explain why the ERAS care is reported to be beneficial for this specific patient group.

Although baby boomer generation accounts for a little more than 15% of the US population, the cohort represents a disproportionate percentage of patients undergoing surgery. As this group continues to age, a multitude of challenges have arisen in health care regarding the safest and most effective means of providing anesthesia services to these patients. Many elderly patients may be exquisitely sensitive to the effects of anesthesia and surgery and may experience cognitive and physical decline before, during, or after hospital admission. In this review article, the authors briefly examine the physiologic processes underlying aging and explore steps necessary to deliver safe, empathetic care.

With the increase in life expectancy in the United States, octogenarians and nonagenarians are more frequently seen in clinical practice. The elderly patients have multiple preexisting comorbidities and are on multiple medications, which can make pain management complex. Moreover, the elderly population often suffers from chronic pain related to degenerative processes, making medical management challenging. In this review, the authors collated available evidence for best practices for pain management in the elderly.

Geriatric Anesthesia

ANESTHESIOLOGY CLINICS

SERIES OF RELATED INTEREST

Critical Care Clinics

THE CLINICS ARE AVAILABLE ONLINE!
Access your subscription at:
www.theclinics.com

Foreword

Geriatric Anesthesia: Ensuring Best Care for Vulnerable Individuals

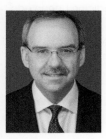

Lee A. Fleisher, MD
Consulting Editor

The COVID-19 pandemic has taught the implications of age on health and resiliency. Even before the pandemic, there was increasing insight on the importance of age on disease and outcomes in the perioperative period. The first article is on perioperative pulmonary complications, which is so relevant in the time of COVID-19. Articles focusing on diseases that are more prevalent in the elderly include perioperative delirium, which is the subject of the Perioperative Brain Health Initiative. Additional topics in which the elderly patient may be associated with increased risks are also discussed, such as ERAS and circulatory support. The editor has also invited two overarching articles on data science and competing priorities in the elderly. Overall, the editor has created an important issue of *Anesthesiology Clinics* to educate us all.

In order to commission an issue on Geriatric Anesthesia, I was able to enlist Shamsuddin Akhtar, MD as the editor. Dr Akhtar is a Professor of Anesthesiology and Pharmacology at Yale University School of Medicine. He is board certified in both Anesthesiology and Critical Care Medicine. Dr Akhtar has conducted multiple outcome studies in the elderly population. He has also completed a textbook entitled "Principles of Geriatric Critical Care" published by Cambridge University. He is Past-President of the Society for Advancement of Geriatric Anesthesia and a board member of the

Anesthesiology Clin 41 (2023) xi–xii
https://doi.org/10.1016/j.anclin.2023.06.002
1932-2275/23/© 2023 Published by Elsevier Inc.

ACE publication by the American Society of Anesthesiology. He has assembled a great group of authors to educate us on geriatric anesthesia.

Lee A. Fleisher, MD
Perelman School of Medicine
at University of Pennsylvania
3400 Spruce Street, Dulles 680
Philadelphia, PA 19104, USA

E-mail address:
Lee.Fleisher@pennmedicine.upenn.edu

Preface
Aging and Growing

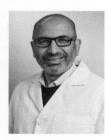

Shamsuddin Akhtar, MD, FASA
Editor

Life expectancy continues to increase in the world. It was 62 years in 1980 and has increased to 73 years in 2020. Life expectancy is around 79 years in the United States, while in Japan it is close to 85 years. Increase in life expectancy is a global phenomenon and is happening both in developed and developing countries. Furthermore, not only is the world population aging, but the proportion of elderly individuals is growing. This increase in the absolute number of elderly patients has significant demographic, social, and economic consequences. By some estimates more than 50% of procedures requiring anesthesia are currently being performed in individuals who are older than 65 years of age and many 80-year-old and older individuals are undergoing procedures that require anesthesia in the operating room and in the nonoperating room settings. This means that most of the practicing anesthesiologists are by default anesthesiologists taking care of geriatric patients, hence should be familiar with special considerations related to elderly patients. This issue of *Anesthesiology Clinics* addresses some of the contemporary issues related to the care of elderly patients. This issue starts by addressing pulmonary complications in the elderly followed by pharmacokinetic and pharmacodynamic changes in the elderly. Delirium continues to be an important area of concern in the perioperative setting, which is addressed in the next article. As technology advances, more and more elderly patients are being considered candidates for receiving mechanical circulatory devices and liver transplantation. The next two articles address these topics. Fluid management, though a mundane topic, is addressed next, as it has significant morbidity implications in the elderly. Proliferation of databases is ubiquitous; hence an article is dedicated to data science and geriatric anesthesia research. Finally, the last three articles deal with areas related to ERAS in elderly patients, efficiency safety, quality, and empathy and pain management in elderly patients. It is hoped that these reviews will update readers on these topics and help practitioners in the perioperative care of elderly patients. Furthermore, the articles address nuances

Anesthesiology Clin 41 (2023) xiii–xiv
https://doi.org/10.1016/j.anclin.2023.06.001
1932-2275/23/© 2023 Published by Elsevier Inc.

anesthesiology.theclinics.com

and highlight gaps in our knowledge regarding perioperative care of elderly patients, which should be an impetus to foster further research in these areas.

Shamsuddin Akhtar, MD, FASA
Department of Anesthesiology and Pharmacology
Critical Care Anesthesiology
Yale School of Medicine
New Haven, CT 06520, USA

E-mail address:
shamsuddin.akhtar@yale.edu

Perioperative Pulmonary Complications in the Older Adults: The Forgotten System

Zyad J. Carr, MD[a],*, Saul Siller, MD[a], Brittany J. McDowell, MD[b]

KEYWORDS

- Postoperative • Pulmonary complications • Perioperative • Anesthesia
- Older Adults • Geriatric

KEY POINTS

- Deleterious physiologic changes associated with aging and the damaging effects of co-morbidities on the pulmonary system, combine to negatively affect perioperative pulmonary outcomes in geriatric populations.
- Older adults populations face a higher risk for perioperative pulmonary complications (PPC) and an increased incidence of frailty that results in increased morbidity, mortality, prolonged hospitalization, institutionalization, and increased health-care expenditures.
- Emerging evidence suggests that a focus on prehabilitative interventions may be effective in reducing PPC.
- Selective identification of preoperative risk factors, procedure-specific risk, and exploiting protective intraoperative and postoperative management strategies can result in reduced incidence of PPC.

BACKGROUND AND DEFINITIONS
Background

Approximately 300 million surgical procedures are performed worldwide annually and surgical volume is increasing each year.[1] Perioperative pulmonary complications (PPC) have long been recognized as an important source of perioperative morbidity and mortality in geriatric populations and its risk factors has been highlighted in perioperative guidelines.[2] Incidence of PPC is approximately 9% and advanced age is a strong predictor for PPC.[3,4] With the projected increase in global geriatric populations (2 billion aged older than 60 years by 2050), surgical and anesthetic techniques will expand the boundaries of safe care in geriatric populations and challenges will be imposed by the increase in PPC.[5]

[a] Department of Anesthesiology, Yale University School of Medicine, TMP-3, 333 Cedar Street, New Haven, CT 06520, USA; [b] Department of Anesthesiology, Intermountain Medical Center, 5121 Cottonwood Street, Murray, UT 84107, USA
* Corresponding author. 333 Cedar Street, TMP-3, New Haven CT 06520.
E-mail address: zyad.carr@yale.edu

Anesthesiology Clin 41 (2023) 531–548
https://doi.org/10.1016/j.anclin.2023.02.005
1932-2275/23/© 2023 Elsevier Inc. All rights reserved.
anesthesiology.theclinics.com

Defining Perioperative Pulmonary Complications

Although a standardized consensus is lacking, most composite definitions of PPC include postoperative pneumonia (POP), persistent or severe postoperative atelectasis, postoperative respiratory failure, pulmonary aspiration, and the acute respiratory distress syndrome.[6] POP remains the primary complication of concern, due to its frequency and associated morbidity and mortality. POP is a serious complication with a 30-day mortality rate of 21%, and a mean increase in length of stay (LOS) by 7 to 9 days.[7,8] POP is estimated to cost the United States health-care system ~US$11.9 billion per year (~US$25,000 per PPC), adding US$717 to the average cost of elective surgery, and may contribute up to 66% of postoperative deaths.[9,10]

PHYSIOLOGIC CHANGES OF THE AGING PULMONARY SYSTEM
Background

An overview of the complex pathophysiology of the aging lung is helpful to understand the increased risk of PPC. Pulmonary function dramatically changes with age and aerobic capacity may decline by upward of 40% between the ages of 24 and 80 years. Declining aerobic capacity is a robust marker of a patient's defense against adverse exertional symptoms.[11] Age-related decline in aerobic capacity is due to progressive loss of muscular, cardiopulmonary, metabolic function and is best quantified by maximal oxygen uptake (Vo_{2max}). After the age of 30 years, Vo_{2max} demonstrates near linear decline of approximately 0.2 to 0.5 mL/min/kg^{-1}/year^{-1} and may accelerate after 40 to 50 years.[12] This accelerated decline in Vo_{2max} is attributable to multiple causes: functional pulmonary dysfunction (pulmonary mechanics, pulmonary vascular function, pulmonary oxygen, and carbon dioxide transport), loss of cardiac function (stroke volume and maximal heart rate decline) and impaired muscle oxidative capacity (muscle-capillary gas exchange, muscle metabolism-mechanical power output coupling). In addition, loss of lung elastic recoil, and subsequent ventilatory limitations also contribute to exercise constraints in geriatric populations. Furthermore, arterial oxygen partial pressure (Pao_2) linearly declines with age reaching a plateau of mean Pao_2 of 73 mm Hg in men and 77 mm Hg in women.[13] These changes are suspected to be mostly related to the aforementioned mechanical ventilatory limitation. However, age-related gas diffusion deficits as demonstrated by age-related decline in diffusing capacity for carbon monoxide (DLCO), physiologic, and shunt-related ventilation/perfusion mismatches have been reported in elderly patients without lung disorders.[14,15] Age-related decline in respiratory muscle mechanics further diminish components measured in pulmonary function tests (PFT) including the loss of lung volumes, increased residual volume, and premature closure of small airways (closing volume).

Implications of Age-Related Cardiopulmonary Decline

Pathophysiological decline is also evident in the pulmonary circulation where pulmonary vascular compliance decreases with age. Decreasing pulmonary vascular compliance is likely a result of reduced left ventricular compliance, that is, diastolic dysfunction, and declining maximal cardiac output, contributing to the erosion of exercise tolerance.[16,17]

Age-Related Neurologic Impairments

Age-related attenuation in central hypoxic and hypercarbic ventilatory responses has been observed but its impact on exercise tolerance is unclear.[18] Older patients have higher prevalence of sleep-disordered breathing, and it likely contributes to a higher risk for mortality.[19] Furthermore, the increasing prevalence of impaired cough reflexes and dysphagia enhances the risk for postoperative aspiration and pneumonia.[20] The culmination of these observed age-related respiratory changes results in reduced clearance of bronchial secretions, alveolar hypoventilation, and a high-risk environment for postoperative respiratory insufficiency and failure.

PULMONARY SYSTEM COMORBIDITIES AND AGING
Impact of Pulmonary Comorbidities: Chronic Obstructive Pulmonary Disease

Chronic obstructive pulmonary disease (COPD), obstructive sleep apnea (OSA), restrictive lung disorders, and cardiovascular diseases all contribute to further deterioration of the pulmonary system in the perioperative period. The prevalence of COPD is estimated to be greater than 11.6% in those aged older than 65 years, with a majority suffering significantly reduced exercise tolerance, increased shortness of breath, and reduced activities of daily living (ADL).[21,22] Perioperatively, COPD is an independent risk factor for the development of postoperative pulmonary infections.[23]

Impact of Pulmonary Comorbidities: Interstitial Lung Disease

Despite their rare prevalence, patients with interstitial lung disease (ILD) are disproportionately represented in the perioperative period. Patients with ILD and its most severe variant, idiopathic pulmonary fibrosis, have higher rates of postoperative acute respiratory worsening (14.2%), acute exacerbation of ILD (5.0%), 30-day POP (9.2%), and 30-day mortality (6%).[24,25]

Impact of Pulmonary Comorbidities: Obstructive Sleep Apnea

Estimates of OSA, central or mixed apnea syndromes, periodic breathing, and nocturnal hypoventilation syndromes in the elderly range as high as 20%. Perioperatively, OSA has been associated with an elevated incidence of PPC, atrial fibrillation, difficult airway, and possibly, postoperative mortality.[19,26] More importantly, increasing age is an independent risk factor for higher severity OSA ($\geq$3 STOP-BANG score) resulting in an increased risk for PPC and longer hospital LOS.[27]

PREOPERATIVE RISK STRATIFICATION
Background

Research continues to further improve the granularity of perioperative risk stratification in geriatric surgical populations. In addition to preoperative procedural and patient risk stratification, quantification of frailty, prehabilitation strategies have expanded opportunities to optimize geriatric patients. Standard preoperative investigations should consider structured interviews, selective use of both cardiopulmonary exercise testing (CPET) and PFT, perioperative risk calculators, and the measurement of frailty severity. Every preoperative evaluation should assess smoking status as even short-term smoking cessation may positively affect PPC.[28–30] Effective interventions for smoking cessation include weekly consultation, beginning 4 to 8 weeks before surgery and use of nicotine replacement therapies.[31] Prehabilitation, utilizing the preoperative time to optimize the physiologic reserve of patients via nutritional and exercise-related intervention, is used to medically optimize identified patients.

Procedural Type is an Important Contributor to Geriatric Postoperative Pulmonary Complications

Perioperative complications are common in oncological surgery, occurring in 18.8% of patients.[32] PPC have been observed in 5.6% of patients undergoing radical cystectomy, resulting in a higher 30-day mortality (17.4% vs 0.7%, $P <$ .001) and longer hospital stay (13 vs 8 days, $P <$ .001). Increasing age (>75 years) was a strong independent predictor for PPC.[33] Regarding the estimated incidence of POP, cardiac and thoracic surgery (3.3%), followed by urologic surgery (1.73%) consisted the highest risk for POP.[34] In a study of 5158 cardiac surgery patients, the cumulative incidence of pneumonia was 2.4% and increasing age (hazard ratio [HR]: 1.02 [95%CI: 1.00, 1.03] $P =$ .05), pre-existing COPD (HR: 2.17 [95%CI: 1.47, 3.21] $P <$ .001), and increasing duration of surgery (HR: 1.38 [95%CI: 1.25, 1.53] $P <$ .001) contributed significantly to the development of POP.[35] POP is a common complication after major lung resection, with an incidence of 25%, is associated with significantly longer intensive care unit stay, hospital stay, and higher risk for in-hospital death.[36] Similarly, there is a 10% incidence of POP after minimally invasive Ivor-Lewis esophagectomy, comprising the primary diagnosis of readmission in 15.4% of all 30-day readmissions.[37,38]

Framing Frailty as a Measure of Fitness for Surgery

Recent findings have observed that advanced age may not be as important as the presence of physiologic frailty, highlighted by the presence of 3 or more of the following characteristics: decreased physical activity, reduced gait velocity, unintentional weight loss, and persistent fatigue.[39] Frailty is defined as a syndrome of declining physiologic reserve that contributes to poor health outcomes, higher risk for institutional care, in-hospital complications, and permanent disability after hospitalization and is best quantified utilizing frailty indices.[40] Although the number of frailty indices have sharply increased, it is important to caution that, with the exception of the Phenotype of Frailty and Frailty index (FI), many are still being validated.[41] A meta-analysis of FI investigating mortality as the primary outcome observed a pooled HR of 1.282 per 0.1 increase in the FI.[42] FI, when compared with age, has been shown to be a superior predictor of in-hospital complications and, possibly, adverse discharge disposition in trauma populations.[43] Furthermore, in a meta-analysis of 683,487 multispecialty surgical patients, frail patients determined by the modified FI (mFI) had a 4.19 higher risk of mortality, faced more major complications (relative risk [RR] 2.03, 95%CI 1.26–3.29; $P =$ .004), wound complications (RR 2.03, 95%CI 1.26–3.29; $P =$ .004) and increased risk of hospital readmission or discharge to skilled nursing facilities.[44] Routine frailty quantification may be a useful addition to perioperative practice, not only to identify those at higher risk for perioperative complications but also for preoperative benefit–risk discussions in geriatric patients.

Quantifying Risk for Postoperative Pulmonary Complications

Numerous tools are available to estimate PPC risk in geriatric populations (**Table 1**).[45] In Arozullah and colleagues risk scoring system, prediction of postoperative nosocomial pneumonia was strongly associated with procedure type and increasing age.[46] The most used and validated scoring system is the Assess Respiratory Risk in Surgical Patients in Catalonia (ARISCAT).[47] The ARISCAT scoring system identified 7 independent risk factors for PPC: age, preoperative anemia, upper abdominal or intrathoracic surgery, increasing length of surgery (>2 hours), preoperative pneumonia (<30 days), low preoperative arterial oxygen saturation, and emergency surgery. Use of these scoring systems may allow for early identification of high-risk patients for the purposes of preoperative intervention, postoperative surveillance, and early, aggressive PPC treatment.

Table 1
Evaluation of perioperative pulmonary risk assessments

ARISCAT Pulmonary Complication Risk Index	Arozullah Respiratory Failure Index	Gupta Postoperative Respiratory Failure Risk
Predicts risk of postoperative pulmonary complications (respiratory failure, infection, effusion, atelectasis, pneumothorax, bronchospasm, aspiration pneumonitis)	Predicts postoperative risk of respiratory failure in elderly patients	Predicts the risk of postoperative mechanical ventilation >48 h or reintubation within 30 d
Age (years)	Age (years)	Procedure type
$\leq$50	$\geq$70	Numerous classes - weighted for severity/ invasiveness
51–80	60–69	
> 80		
Preoperative SpO_2		ASA class
$\geq$96%		Class I–V
91%–95%		
$\leq$90%		
Other clinical risk factors	Other clinical risk factors	Other clinical risk factors
Respiratory infection in the last month	Partially or fully dependent functional status	Emergency case
Preoperative anemia with Hgb $\leq$10 g/dL	History of COPD	Sepsis
Emergency surgery	Emergency surgery	Preoperative SIRS
Surgical incision	Type of surgery	Preoperative septic shock
Upper abdominal	Abdominal aortic aneurysm	Preoperative sepsis
Intrathoracic	Thoracic	None
	NSGY, upper abdominal, peripheral vascular	Functional status
Duration of surgery	Neck	Totally dependent
<2 h	Laboratory findings	Partially dependent
2–3 h	Albumin <3.0 g/dL	Totally independent
>3 h	BUN >30 mg/dL	
Estimated risk probability of pulmonary complication	Estimated risk probability of respiratory failure	Estimated risk probability of respiratory failure
0–25 points: Low risk: 1.6%	Class 1: $\leq$10 points: 0.5%	Postoperative respiratory failure risk, % = ex/ (1 + ex)
26–44 points: Intermediate risk: 13.3%	Class 2: 11–19 points: 1.8%	*Where x = −1.7397 + sum of the selected variables

(*continued on next page*)

Table 1 *(continued)*		
ARISCAT Pulmonary Complication Risk Index	Arozullah Respiratory Failure Index	Gupta Postoperative Respiratory Failure Risk
45–123 points: High risk: 42.1%	Class 3: 20–27 points: 4.2%	
	Class 4: 28–40 points: 10.1%	
	Class 5: >40 points: 26.6%	

Abbreviations: ASA, American Society Of Anesthesiologists Physical Status; BUN, blood urea nitrogen; NSGY, neurosurgery; SIRS, systemic inflammatory response; SpO_2, oxygen saturation.

Evidence-Based Guidance for Special Preoperative Investigations

Certain procedures or comorbid conditions may benefit from more extensive preoperative pulmonary testing. In patients with COPD or asthma, spirometry values may identify a reversible obstructive component that can be targeted for preoperative medical optimization.[48] The American College of Chest Physicians recommend that patients with a forced expiratory volume (1 second) or DLCO less than 40% of predicted value receive CPET for further extrapolation of perioperative risk before lung resection. A Vo_{2max} less than 15 mL/kg/min is strongly suggestive of increased perioperative complications, including death.[49] CPET referral, although limited by availability and cost, has been studied in preoperative risk stratification in noncardiothoracic surgery such as colorectal, abdominal aortic aneurysmal repair, and general abdominal surgery. Vo_{2max} and anaerobic thresholds have been identified for 90-day to 3-year survival, ICU admission, increasing LOS, and other major cardiopulmonary morbidity.[50,51] Given the increasing incidence of dysphagia with age, preoperative evaluation of swallowing reflexes may minimize the incidence of aspiration pneumonitis for select surgical procedures. Preoperative swallowing evaluation before esophagectomy both decreased the incidence of aspiration, and reliably predicted POP in this population.[52] Identifying patients with subacute or undertreated pneumonia before their surgery should be emphasized in the preoperative evaluation. In a cohort of more than 7000 geriatric hip fracture patients, preoperative pneumonia was found in 1.2% and was associated with higher rates of serious adverse events and death (RR = 2.08).[53] A retrospective cohort study of the NSQIP database found a preoperative pneumonia incidence of 0.5% among all age groups presenting for elective or emergency surgery and found higher composite morbidity (odds ratio [OR] 1.68 (95% CI: 1.58–1.79) and mortality (OR: 1.37 [95% CI: 1.26–1.48]) in this patient population.[54]

PREHABILITATION
Deconditioning in Geriatric Populations is Underrecognized

Deconditioning in perioperative patients has been observed to increase the risk for PPC.[55,56] Recent clinical data have demonstrated the efficacy of preoperative identification, quantification and treatment of sarcopenia and preoperative nutritional status as a method to reduce perioperative morbidity and mortality. Quantification of sarcopenia, defined as low muscle strength and quantity, and low nutritional status utilizing markers such as the controlling nutritional status (CONUT) score, skeletal muscle index, or creatinine/cystatin C (CysC) ratio may be useful in identifying high-risk patients in the perioperative time period.[57–63]

Prehabilitation May Reduce Perioperative Morbidity

Clinical investigations have demonstrated moderate-to-strong efficacy with even minimal efforts in exercise prehabilitation with or without nutritional supplementation.

Patients randomized to receive a short preoperative program of moderate aerobic exercises, resistance exercises, nutritional counseling, and protein supplementation demonstrated improvements in preoperative functional capacity.[64] In high-risk patients presenting for elective major abdominal surgery, prehabilitation focused predominantly on high-intensity exercise, inspiratory muscle training, or physiotherapy resulted in enhanced aerobic capacity and decreased major postoperative complications including PPC.[65–68] Prehabilitation, although findings have been encouraging, remains in its development stage. Clinical trials have solidified its role in geriatric preoperative optimization, with evidence of reduction of perioperative morbidity, mortality, and reduction of PPC.[69–71] Globally, there are over 266 ongoing clinical trials of prehabilitation in older populations. The results of these trials should further address important questions regarding timing, specific strategies, and clinical outcomes in the perioperative time period.

INTRAOPERATIVE STRATEGIES
Background

Adults aged 65 years and older have been identified as an important population for specialized perioperative guidelines but have been predominately procedure or co-morbidity-specific.[72–75] General intraoperative recommendations include the consideration of regional anesthesia for the reduction of postoperative complications and reduction of postoperative pain, minimization of opioids to reduce delirium, prevention of pressure-related injuries, minimization of intraoperative fluid administration, close hemodynamic management, and ensuring timely administration of home medications. Careful attention to polypharmacy and avoidance of potentially deleterious medications may reduce the risk of compromised respiratory mechanics and impaired protective airway reflexes.[76]

Specific Intraoperative Recommendation: Choice of Anesthetic

Exhaustive systematic trials assessing epidural or spinal anesthesia have demonstrated RR reduction of POP (39%), overall mortality and major complications when compared with general endotracheal anesthesia.[77] Newer analysis has been less positive for regional anesthesia, and this remains an area of active investigation.

Specific Intraoperative Recommendation: Neuromuscular Blockade

Choice of neuromuscular blockade and its reversal remains an important opportunity in reducing impaired respiratory mechanics in the immediate postoperative time period.[78] Sugammadex (Bridion™, Merck, Rahway, NJ), a novel cyclodextrin and first in class selective relaxant binding agent, has revolutionized nondepolarizing neuromuscular blockade reversal and has been observed to reduce the incidence of PPC.[79,80]

Specific Intraoperative Recommendation: Ventilator Strategies

Clinical trials of intraoperative low-tidal volume ventilation and reduced mechanical ventilator driving pressure have observed reductions in postoperative noninvasive ventilation, endotracheal intubation for acute respiratory failure, composite PPC, improved postoperative PFT, and reduced clinical pulmonary infection scores.[81–83] In contrast, a meta-analysis of intraoperative high positive end-expiratory pressure (PEEP) or recruitment maneuvers during low-tidal volume ventilation did not demonstrate a reduction in PPC.[84]

Table 2
Selected references on best practice regarding the prevention of PPC in geriatric populations

Phase	Author Year	Summary	Key Finding
Preoperative			
	Kojima G et al,[42] 2018	Frailty measured by FI is a significant predictor of mortality	HR per 0.01 FI increase = 1.039, $P < .001$
	Canet J et al,[47] 2010	7 factors are independently associated with postoperative pulmonary complications: low preoperative oxygen saturation, acute respiratory infection (<30d), age, preoperative anemia, surgical duration >2h, upper abdominal/thoracic/emergency surgery	Risk index demonstrated an AUC 88% (95% CI, 84%–93%)
	Moran J et al,[50] 2016	Systematic review. Preliminary CPET thresholds for an increased risk of postoperative complications	VO_2peak <15 mL.kg^{-1}.min^{-1} associated with decreased 90-d survival after AAA repair
	Steffens D et al,[51] 2021	Systematic review and meta-analysis. Preoperative CPET predicts postoperative outcomes	Strong association between higher VO_2 peak and absence of postoperative complication including PPC
	Lugg ST et al, 2017	Prospective observational of smoking status and lung resection surgery	Current smokers have higher rate of PPC (22% vs 2%, $P = .004$) ex-smokers <6 wk had lower rates of PPC
	Lindstrom D et al,[29] 2008	RCT of smoking cessation therapy with individual therapy and nicotine substitution 4 wk before surgery	Overall complication rate (41% vs 21% intervention group). Small study.
	Kim HJ et al,[58] 2021	Assessment of creatinine/cystatin C ratio in a cohort of elderly patients undergoing cardiac surgery	A 10-unit increase of creatinine/cystatin ratio was associated with lower risk of PPC (OR 0.80, 95% CI 0.69–92, $P = .001$) Optimal cut-off was 89.5
	Kuroda D et al,[59] 2017	Retrospective Analysis. Preoperative CONUT comparison of CONUT high (>4) vs CONUT low (<3) patients who underwent curative gastric cancer resection	High CONUT score was a highly accurate predictor of nutritional status as well as long-term survival

Prehabilitation		
Moran J et al,[50] 2016	Systematic review and meta-analysis. Prehabilitation (inspiratory muscle training, aerobic exercises, resistance training) reduces postoperative complications	OR: 0.59 (95% CI: 0.38, 0.91, $P = .03$). Methodologic quality of studies was low
Gillis C et al,[64] 2014	Parallel-arm single-blind clinical trial. Randomized to either moderate aerobic and resistance exercises, nutrition counseling, or placebo 4 wk before surgery	Higher percentage of prehabilitation group recovered to baseline exercise capacity (84 vs 62% adjusted $P = .049$)
Barberan-Garcia A et al,[65] 2018	Randomized, blinded, clinical trial. Intervention arm received high-intensity endurance training and counseling	Intervention group reduced postoperative complications (OR 0.5, 95% CI: 0.3–0.8; $P = .001$)
Hughes MJ et al,[70] 2019	Meta-analysis of 15 RCT analyzing prehabilitation before major abdominal surgery	Significant reduction in pulmonary morbidity (OR 0.4 95% CI 0.23–0.68; $P = .0007$)
Intraoperative		
Kheterpal S et al,[80] 2020	Retrospective, matching comparative cohort comparing PPC in patients receiving sugammadex vs neostigmine for neuromuscular blockade reversal	Sugammadex was associated with a 30% reduction in PPC (adjusted OR: 0.7, 95%CI, 0.63–0.77) and postoperative pneumonia (adjusted OR 0.53, 95% CI, 0.44–0.62)
Neto AS et al,[82] 2016	Meta-analysis of 17 randomized clinical trial of protective intraoperative lung ventilation strategies	Increased driving pressure or PEEP that raised driving pressure was associated with more PPC (OR 3.11, 95% CI 1.39–6.96; $P = .006$)
Postoperative		
Zarbock A et al,[94] 2009	Randomized clinical trial of nasal CPAP compared to standard treatment	Hypoxemia, pneumonia and reintubation rates were reduced ($P = .03$)
Ferreyra GP et al,[95] 2008	Meta-analysis. 9 randomized controlled trials of CPAP vs standard therapy after major abdominal surgery	CPAP reduced the of PPC (risk ratio 0.66, 95% CI, 0.52–0.85)
Cassidy MR et al,[102] 2013	Before-after trial. Implementation of the I COUGH multidisciplinary pulmonary care bundle	Incidence of pneumonia fell from 2.6% to 1.6% after implementation of I-COUGH resulting in a risk-adjusted OR of 2.1–1.31
Caparelli ML et al,[101] 2019	Before-after trial. Implementation of an oral care bundle in elective cardiac surgery patients	Reported incidence of postoperative pneumonia dropped from 0.8 to 0% with a risk-adjusted OR from 1.17 to 0.33

Abbreviations: AUC, area under the curve; CI, confidence interval; CONUT, controlling nutritional status score; CPET, cardiopulmonary exercise testing; FI, frailty index; PPC, postoperative pulmonary complications; RCT, randomized controlled trial; VO2peak, maximal oxygen consumption.

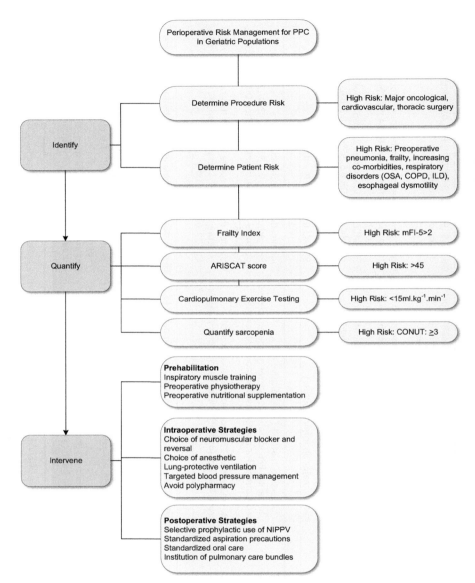

Fig. 1. A visual representation of clinical best practice for mitigating PPC in geriatric popu-lations. ARISCAT, Assess Respiratory Risk in Surgical Patients in Catalonia; CONUT, Control-ling Nutritional Status Score; COPD, chronic obstructive pulmonary disease; ILD, interstitial lung disease; mFI, modified Frailty Index; NIPPV, noninvasive positive pressure ventilation; OSA, obstructive sleep apnea; PPC, postoperative pulmonary complications.

Specific Intraoperative Recommendation: Individualized Blood Pressure Management

Individualized systolic blood pressure management, aiming to adhere to patients' pre-operative blood pressure, significantly reduced 30-day pneumonia and sepsis.[85]

These simple intraoperative measures, when aggregated, may represent an opportunity for improved perioperative outcomes.

POSTOPERATIVE STRATEGIES
Background

Traditional evidence-based consensus recommendations for PPC have focused on chest physiotherapy, incentive spirometry, programs of early mobilization, and standardization of aspiration precautions. New evidence has demonstrated the efficacy of noninvasive positive pressure ventilation (NIPPV) in reducing PPC.

Postoperative Strategies: Pulmonary Hygiene Measures

Traditional measures such as postoperative incentive spirometry, chest physiotherapy, and deep breathing exercises have not demonstrated clear benefit in the reduction of PPC. In a 2001 systematic review of these interventions, the authors suggested many of the included studies were methodologically flawed, although incentive spirometry demonstrated modest benefit following abdominal surgery.[86,87] Similarly, a 2011 review found a lack of evidence to specifically support the routine use of postoperative incentive spirometry but some efficacy for use after gastrointestinal surgery.[88]

Postoperative Strategies: Nutritional Support

Focused postoperative nutritional support remains a source of ongoing research, given the association of PPC with preoperative malnutrition but strong support has not been forthcoming.[89,90]

Postoperative Strategies: Noninvasive Positive Pressure Respiratory Support

More promising evidence has been displayed with the use of noninvasive positive pressure devices. Preemptive use of noninvasive pulmonary ventilation, either continuous positive airway pressure (CPAP) or high-flow nasal cannula, is effective in minimizing postoperative atelectasis and volume overload-related respiratory insufficiency. NIPPV seems to be important adjunct in reducing PPC, particularly in patients with morbid obesity, upper abdominal surgery, or history of OSA.[91] Prophylactic, rather than rescue, use of NIPPV may maximize its benefits and the overall consensus is that NIPPV use improves survival in postoperative acute care settings.[92,93] A clinical trial of postoperative prophylactic NIPPV in patients undergoing cardiac surgery, a known cause of significant postoperative atelectasis, observed a significant reduction in the incidence of pulmonary complications, including pneumonia, reintubation, and readmission to the ICU.[94] Other studies have further supported the benefit of NIPPV in the prevention of PPC, including atelectasis, pneumonia, and as a potential alternative to reintubation.[95–98] Due to the high prevalence of PPC, care bundles have come into widespread use to provide consistent effort, magnify smaller incremental benefits of individual interventions, and reduce barriers to implementation. Most care bundles have focused on oral care, smoking cessation, nutritional support, incentive spirometry, physical therapy, respiratory exercises, and have demonstrated moderate-to-high efficacy in reducing PPC.[99–102]

SUMMARY

With a rapidly aging population and increasing global surgical volumes, managing the risk of PPC has become an important focus for quality improvement in health care **(Table 2)**. Improvements in preoperative identification of high-risk comorbidities and surgical procedures, frailty assessment, and pneumonia risk stratification tools have led to an improved PPC risk profiling (**Fig. 1**). Prehabilitation interventions such as nutritional supplementation, physiotherapy, and inspiratory muscle training seem to have a promising role in optimizing geriatric patients for surgery and potentially reducing PPC. Intraoperative improvements in neuromuscular blockade reversal, lung-protective ventilation strategies, and targeted blood pressure management have shown promise in reducing PPC. Clinical evidence continues to expand the postoperative role of NIPPV, oral care, early aspiration evaluation, and pulmonary care bundles to reduce PPC. Furthermore, traditional measures such as incentive spirometry and postoperative physiotherapy have shown limited benefit, providing opportunity to reduce health-care costs. Development of geriatric-specific enhanced recovery after surgery protocols may further mitigate risk and optimize outcomes for this high-risk patient population. We are optimistic that ongoing incremental improvements in clinical interventions will further reduce morbidity, mortality, and health-care cost associated with the age-old dilemma of PPC in geriatric populations.

CLINICS CARE POINTS

- Despite incremental improvements in perioperative care, geriatric patients face significant morbidity and mortality from PPC.
- Focused preoperative PPC risk stratification by identifying patient and procedure-specific risk, frailty quantification, and selective preoperative testing will assist in modeling realistic assessments of postoperative outcome.
- Recent developments in prehabilitation, intraoperative strategies, and postoperative respiratory support coupled with the success of pulmonary care bundles have provided real reductions in PPC.

DISCLOSURE

The authors have nothing to disclose.

REFERENCES

1. Weiser TG, Haynes AB, Molina G, et al. Estimate of the global volume of surgery in 2012: an assessment supporting improved health outcomes. Lancet (London, England) 2015;385(Suppl 2):S11.
2. Chow WB, Rosenthal RA, Merkow RP, et al. Optimal Preoperative Assessment of the Geriatric Surgical Patient: A Best Practices Guideline from the American College of Surgeons National Surgical Quality Improvement Program and the American Geriatrics Society. J Am Coll Surg 2012;215(4):453–66.
3. Meguid RA, Bronsert MR, Juarez-Colunga E, et al. Surgical Risk Preoperative Assessment System (SURPAS): III. Accurate Preoperative Prediction of 8 Adverse Outcomes Using 8 Predictor Variables. Annals of surgery 2016; 264(1):23–31.
4. Madsen HJ, Meguid RA, Bronsert MR, et al. Associations between preoperative risks of postoperative complications: Results of an analysis of 4.8 Million ACS-NSQIP patients. Am J Surg 2021;223(6):1172–8.
5. Sander M, Oxlund B, Jespersen A, et al. The challenges of human population ageing. Age Ageing 2015;44(2):185–7.

6. Abbott TEF, Fowler AJ, Pelosi P, et al. A systematic review and consensus definitions for standardised end-points in perioperative medicine: pulmonary complications. British journal of anaesthesia 2018;120(5):1066–79.
7. Hall JC, Tarala RA, Hall JL, et al. A multivariate analysis of the risk of pulmonary complications after laparotomy. Chest 1991;99(4):923–7.
8. Rello J, Ollendorf DA, Oster G, et al. Epidemiology and outcomes of ventilator-associated pneumonia in a large US database. Chest 2002;122(6):2115–21.
9. Fleisher LA, Linde-Zwirble WT. Incidence, outcome, and attributable resource use associated with pulmonary and cardiac complications after major small and large bowel procedures. Perioper Med (Lond) 2014;3:7.
10. Linde-Zwirble W, Bloom J, Mecca R, et al. Postoperative pulmonary complications in adult elective surgery patients in the US: severity, outcomes and resources use. Crit Care 2010;14(1):1–2.
11. Roman MA, Rossiter HB, Casaburi R. Exercise, ageing and the lung. Eur Respir J 2016;48(5):1471–86.
12. Fleg JL, Morrell CH, Bos AG, et al. Accelerated longitudinal decline of aerobic capacity in healthy older adults. Circulation 2005;112(5):674–82.
13. Hardie JA, Vollmer WM, Buist AS, et al. Reference values for arterial blood gases in the elderly. Chest 2004;125(6):2053–60.
14. McClaran SR, Babcock MA, Pegelow DF, et al. Longitudinal effects of aging on lung function at rest and exercise in healthy active fit elderly adults. Journal of applied physiology (Bethesda, Md 1985) 1995;78(5):1957–68.
15. Cardús J, Burgos F, Diaz O, et al. Increase in pulmonary ventilation-perfusion inequality with age in healthy individuals. Am J Respir Crit Care Med 1997; 156(2 Pt 1):648–53.
16. Bhella PS, Hastings JL, Fujimoto N, et al. Impact of lifelong exercise "dose" on left ventricular compliance and distensibility. J Am Coll Cardiol 2014;64(12): 1257–66.
17. Hieda M, Howden E, Shibata S, et al. Impact of Lifelong Exercise Training Dose on Ventricular-Arterial Coupling. Circulation 2018;138(23):2638–47.
18. Janssens JP. Aging of the respiratory system: impact on pulmonary function tests and adaptation to exertion. Clin Chest Med 2005;26(3):469–84, vi-vii.
19. Janssens JP, Pautex S, Hilleret H, et al. Sleep disordered breathing in the elderly. Aging (Milano) 2000;12(6):417–29.
20. Marik PE, Kaplan D. Aspiration pneumonia and dysphagia in the elderly. Chest 2003;124(1):328–36.
21. Incalzi RA, Scarlata S, Pennazza G, et al. Chronic Obstructive Pulmonary Disease in the elderly. Eur J Intern Med 2014;25(4):320–8.
22. CfDCa Prevention. Chronic obstructive pulmonary disease among adults–United States, 2011. MMWR Morb Mortal Wkly Rep 2012;61(46):938–43.
23. Conde M, Lawrence V. Postoperative pulmonary infections. BMJ Clin Evid 2008; 2008:1–18.
24. McDowell BJ, Karamchandani K, Lehman EB, et al. Perioperative risk factors in patients with idiopathic pulmonary fibrosis: a historical cohort study. Canadian Journal of Anesthesia-Journal Canadien D Anesthesie 2021;68(1):81–91.
25. Carr ZJ, Yan L, Chavez-Duarte J, et al. Perioperative Management of Patients with Idiopathic Pulmonary Fibrosis Undergoing Noncardiac Surgery: A Narrative Review. Int J Gen Med 2022;15:2087–100.
26. Opperer M, Cozowicz C, Bugada D, et al. Does Obstructive Sleep Apnea Influence Perioperative Outcome? A Qualitative Systematic Review for the Society of

Anesthesia and Sleep Medicine Task Force on Preoperative Preparation of Patients with Sleep-Disordered Breathing. Anesth Analg 2016;122(5):1321–34.

27. Pereira H, Xara D, Mendonca J, et al. Patients with a high risk for obstructive sleep apnea syndrome: postoperative respiratory complications. Rev Port Pneumol 2013;19(4):144–51.

28. Napolitano MA, Rosenfeld ES, Chen SW, et al. Impact of Timing of Smoking Cessation on 30-Day Outcomes in Veterans Undergoing Lobectomy for Cancer. Semin Thorac Cardiovasc Surg 2021;33(3):860–8.

29. Lindstrom D, Azodi OS, Wadis A, et al. Effects of a Perioperative Smoking Cessation Intervention on Postoperative Complications A Randomized Trial. Annals of surgery 2008;248(5):739–45.

30. Mills E, Eyawo O, Lockhart I, et al. Smoking Cessation Reduces Postoperative Complications: A Systematic Review and Meta-analysis. Am J Med 2011; 124(2):144–U144.

31. Thomsen T, Villebro N, Moller AM. Interventions for preoperative smoking cessation. Cochrane Database Syst Rev 2010;7.

32. Liu JB, Berian JR, Liu Y, et al. Trends in perioperative outcomes of hospitals performing major cancer surgery. J Surg Oncol 2018;118(4):694–703.

33. Xia L, Taylor BL, Guzzo TJ. Characteristics and Associated Factors of Postoperative Pulmonary Complications in Patients Undergoing Radical Cystectomy for Bladder Cancer: A National Surgical Quality Improvement Program Study. Clin Genitourin Cancer 2017;15(6):661–9.

34. Chughtai M, Gwam CU, Khlopas A, et al. The Incidence of Postoperative Pneumonia in Various Surgical Subspecialties: A Dual Database Analysis. Surg Technol Int 2017;30:45–51.

35. Ailawadi G, Chang HL, O'Gara PT, et al. Pneumonia after cardiac surgery: Experience of the National Institutes of Health/Canadian Institutes of Health Research Cardiothoracic Surgical Trials Network. J Thorac Cardiovasc Surg 2017;153(6): 1384–1391 e1383.

36. Schussler O, Alifano M, Dermine H, et al. Postoperative pneumonia after major lung resection. Am J Respir Crit Care Med 2006;173(10):1161–9.

37. Casas MA, Angeramo CA, Bras Harriott C, et al. Surgical outcomes after totally minimally invasive Ivor Lewis esophagectomy. A systematic review and meta-analysis. Eur J Surg Oncol 2022;48(3):473–81.

38. Park SY, Kim DJ, Byun GE. Incidence and risk factors of readmission after esophagectomy for esophageal cancer. J Thorac Dis 2019;11(11):4700–7.

39. Fried LP, Tangen CM, Walston J, et al. Frailty in older adults: evidence for a phenotype. Journals of Gerontology Series A, Biological sciences and medical sciences 2001;56(3):M146–56.

40. Wu KY, Gouda P, Wang X, et al. Association of Frailty, Age, Socioeconomic Status, and Type of Surgery With Perioperative Outcomes in Patients Undergoing Noncardiac Surgery. JAMA Netw Open 2022;5(7):e2224625.

41. Bouillon K, Kivimaki M, Hamer M, et al. Measures of frailty in population-based studies: an overview. BMC Geriatr 2013;13.

42. Kojima G, Iliffe S, Walters K. Frailty index as a predictor of mortality: a systematic review and meta-analysis. Age Ageing 2018;47(2):193–200.

43. Joseph B, Pandit V, Zangbar B, et al. Superiority of Frailty Over Age in Predicting Outcomes Among Geriatric Trauma Patients A Prospective Analysis. JAMA surgery 2014;149(8):766–72.

44. Panayi AC, Orkaby AR, Sakthivel D, et al. Impact of frailty on outcomes in surgical patients: A systematic review and meta-analysis. Am J Surg 2019; 218(2):393–400.
45. Gupta H, Gupta PK, Fang X, et al. Development and Validation of a Risk Calculator Predicting Postoperative Respiratory Failure. Chest 2011;140(5):1207–15.
46. Arozullah AM, Khuri SF, Henderson WG, et al. Development and validation of a multifactorial risk index for predicting postoperative pneumonia after major noncardiac surgery. Ann Intern Med 2001;135(10):847–57.
47. Canet J, Gallart L, Gomar C, et al. Prediction of Postoperative Pulmonary Complications in a Population-based Surgical Cohort. Anesthesiology 2010;113(6): 1338–50.
48. Bernstein WK. Pulmonary function testing. Curr Opin Anaesthesiol 2012; 25(1):11–6.
49. Colice GL, Shafazand S, Griffin JP, et al. Physiologic evaluation of the patient with lung cancer being considered for resectional surgery: ACCP evidenced-based clinical practice guidelines (2nd edition). Chest 2007;132(3 Suppl): 161s–77s.
50. Moran J, Wilson F, Guinan E, et al. Role of cardiopulmonary exercise testing as a risk-assessment method in patients undergoing intra-abdominal surgery: a systematic review. British journal of anaesthesia 2016;116(2):177–91.
51. Steffens D, Ismail H, Denehy L, et al. Preoperative Cardiopulmonary Exercise Test Associated with Postoperative Outcomes in Patients Undergoing Cancer Surgery: A Systematic Review and Meta-Analyses. Ann Surg Oncol 2021; 28(12):7120–46.
52. Berry MF, Atkins BZ, Tong BC, et al. A comprehensive evaluation for aspiration after esophagectomy reduces the incidence of postoperative pneumonia. J Thorac Cardiovasc Surg 2010;140(6):1266–71.
53. Patterson JT, Bohl DD, Basques BA, et al. Does Preoperative Pneumonia Affect Complications of Geriatric Hip Fracture Surgery? Am J Orthop (Belle Mead NJ) 2017;46(3):E177–85.
54. Jamali S, Dagher M, Bilani N, et al. The Effect of Preoperative Pneumonia on Postsurgical Mortality and Morbidity: A NSQIP Analysis. World J Surg 2018; 42(9):2763–72.
55. Canet J, Mazo V. Postoperative pulmonary complications. Minerva Anestesiol 2010;76(2):138–43.
56. Bohl DD, Sershon RA, Saltzman BM, et al. Incidence, Risk Factors, and Clinical Implications of Pneumonia After Surgery for Geriatric Hip Fracture. J Arthroplasty 2018;33(5):1552.
57. Iseki Y, Shibutani M, Maeda K, et al. Impact of the Preoperative Controlling Nutritional Status (CONUT) Score on the Survival after Curative Surgery for Colorectal Cancer. PLoS One 2015;10(7).
58. Kim HJ, Kim HB, Kim HY, et al. Associations of creatinine/cystatin C ratio and postoperative pulmonary complications in elderly patients undergoing off-pump coronary artery bypass surgery: a retrospective study. Sci Rep 2021; 11(1):16881.
59. Kuroda D, Sawayama H, Kurashige J, et al. Controlling Nutritional Status (CONUT) score is a prognostic marker for gastric cancer patients after curative resection. Gastric Cancer 2018;21(2):204–12.
60. Tokunaga R, Sakamoto Y, Nakagawa S, et al. CONUT: a novel independent predictive score for colorectal cancer patients undergoing potentially curative resection. Int J Colorectal Dis 2017;32(1):99–106.

61. Lieffers JR, Bathe OF, Fassbender K, et al. Sarcopenia is associated with post-operative infection and delayed recovery from colorectal cancer resection surgery. Br J Cancer 2012;107(6):931–6.

62. Moisey LL, Mourtzakis M, Cotton BA, et al. Skeletal muscle predicts ventilator-free days, ICU-free days, and mortality in elderly ICU patients. Crit Care 2013;17(5).

63. Harimoto N, Shirabe K, Yamashita YI, et al. Sarcopenia as a predictor of prognosis in patients following hepatectomy for hepatocellular carcinoma. Br J Surg 2013;100(11):1523–30.

64. Gillis C, Li C, Lee L, et al. Prehabilitation versus Rehabilitation A Randomized Control Trial in Patients Undergoing Colorectal Resection for Cancer. Anesthesiology 2014;121(5):937–47.

65. Barberan-Garcia A, Ubre M, Roca J, et al. Personalised Prehabilitation in High-risk Patients Undergoing Elective Major Abdominal Surgery: A Randomized Blinded Controlled Trial. Annals of surgery 2018;267(1):50–6.

66. Minnella EM, Awasthi R, Loiselle SE, et al. Effect of Exercise and Nutrition Prehabilitation on Functional Capacit in Esophagogastric ancer Surgery A Randomized Clinical Trial. JAMA surgery 2018;153(12):1081–9.

67. Boden I, Skinner EH, Browning L, et al. Preoperative physiotherapy for the prevention of respiratory complications after upper abdominal surgery: pragmatic, double blinded, multicentre randomised controlled trial. BMJ Br Med J (Clin Res Ed) 2018;360.

68. Boden I, Denehy L. Respiratory Prehabilitation for the Prevention of Postoperative Pulmonary Complications after Major Surgery. Current Anesthesiology Reports 2022;12(1):44–58.

69. Jones LW, Peddle CJ, Eves ND, et al. Effects of presurgical exercise training on cardiorespiratory fitness among patients undergoing thoracic surgery for malignant lung lesions. Cancer 2007;110(3):590–8.

70. Hughes MJ, Hackney RJ, Lamb PJ, et al. Prehabilitation Before Major Abdominal Surgery: A Systematic Review and Meta-analysis. World J Surg 2019; 43(7):1661–8.

71. Hijazi Y, Gondal U, Aziz O. A systematic review of prehabilitation programs in abdominal cancer surgery. Int J Surg 2017;39:156–62.

72. Mohanty S, Rosenthal RA, Russell MM, et al. Optimal Perioperative Management of the Geriatric Patient: A Best Practices Guideline from the American College of Surgeons NSQIP and the American Geriatrics Society. J Am Coll Surg 2016;222(5):930–47.

73. Alvarez-Nebreda ML, Bentov N, Urman RD, et al. Recommendations for Preoperative Management of Frailty from the Society for Perioperative Assessment and Quality Improvement (SPAQI). J Clin Anesth 2018;47:33–42.

74. Beaupre LA, Jones CA, Saunders LD, et al. Best practices for elderly hip fracture patients - A systematic overview of the evidence. J Gen Intern Med 2005; 20(11):1019–25.

75. Berian JR, Rosenthal RA, Baker TL, et al. Hospital Standards to Promote Optimal Surgical Care of the Older Adult A Report From the Coalition for Quality in Geriatric Surgery. Annals of surgery 2018;267(2):280–90.

76. American Geriatrics Society 2019 Updated AGS Beers Criteria® for Potentially Inappropriate Medication Use in Older Adults. J Am Geriatr Soc 2019;67(4): 674–94.

77. Rodgers A, Walker N, Schug S, et al. Reduction of postoperative mortality and morbidity with epidural or spinal anaesthesia: results from overview of randomised trials. BMJ Br Med J (Clin Res Ed) 2000;321(7275):1493–7.
78. Murphy GS, Szokol JW, Marymont JH, et al. Residual neuromuscular blockade and critical respiratory events in the postanesthesia care unit. Anesth Analg 2008;107(1):130–7.
79. Khuenl-Brady KS, Wattwil M, Vanacker BF, et al. Sugammadex Provides Faster Reversal of Vecuronium-Induced Neuromuscular Blockade Compared with Neostigmine: A Multicenter, Randomized, Controlled Trial. Anesth Analg 2010; 110(1):64–73.
80. Kheterpal S, Vaughn MT, Dubovoy TZ, et al. Sugammadex versus Neostigmine for Reversal of Neuromuscular Blockade and Postoperative Pulmonary Complications (STRONGER): A Multicenter Matched Cohort Analysis. Anesthesiology 2020;132(6):1371–81.
81. Futier E, Constantin J-M, Paugam-Burtz C, et al. A Trial of Intraoperative Low-Tidal-Volume Ventilation in Abdominal Surgery. N Engl J Med 2013;369(5): 428–37.
82. Neto AS, Hemmes SNT, Barbas CSV, et al. Association between driving pressure and development of postoperative pulmonary complications in patients undergoing mechanical ventilation for general anaesthesia: a meta-analysis of individual patient data. Lancet Respir Med 2016;4(4):272–80.
83. Severgnini P, Selmo G, Lanza C, et al. Protective Mechanical Ventilation during General Anesthesia for Open Abdominal Surgery Improves Postoperative Pulmonary Function. Anesthesiology 2013;118(6):1307–21.
84. Campos NS, Bluth T, Hemmes SNT, et al. Intraoperative positive end-expiratory pressure and postoperative pulmonary complications: a patient-level meta-analysis of three randomised clinical trials. British journal of anaesthesia 2022; 128(6):1040–51.
85. Futier E, Lefrant JY, Guinot PG, et al. Effect of Individualized vs Standard Blood Pressure Management Strategies on Postoperative Organ Dysfunction Among High-Risk Patients Undergoing Major Surgery: A Randomized Clinical Trial. JAMA 2017;318(14):1346–57.
86. Overend TJ, Anderson CM, Lucy SD, et al. The effect of incentive spirometry on postoperative pulmonary complications - A systematic review. Chest 2001; 120(3):971–8.
87. Reeve JC, Nicol K, Stiller K, et al. Does physiotherapy reduce the incidence of postoperative pulmonary complications following pulmonary resection via open thoracotomy? A preliminary randomised single-blind clinical trial. Eur J Cardio Thorac Surg 2010;37(5):1158–66.
88. Restrepo RD, Wettstein R, Wittnebel L, et al. Incentive Spirometry: 2011. Respir Care 2011;56(10):1600–4.
89. Koretz RL, Avenell A, Lipman TO, et al. Does enteral nutrition affect clinical outcome? A systematic review of the randomized trials. Am J Gastroenterol 2007;102(2):412–29 [quiz: 468].
90. Avenell A, Smith TO, Curtain JP, et al. Nutritional supplementation for hip fracture aftercare in older people. Cochrane Database Syst Rev 2016;11(11): Cd001880.
91. Cereda M, Neligan PJ, Reed AJ. Noninvasive respiratory support in the perioperative period. Current Opinion in Anesthesiology 2013;26(2):134–40.

92. Cabrini L, Landoni G, Oriani A, et al. Noninvasive Ventilation and Survival in Acute Care Settings: A Comprehensive Systematic Review and Metaanalysis of Randomized Controlled Trials. Crit Care Med 2015;43(4):880–8.

93. Neligan PJ, Malhotra G, Fraser M, et al. Continuous Positive Airway Pressure via the Boussignac System Immediately after Extubation Improves Lung Function in Morbidly Obese Patients with Obstructive Sleep Apnea Undergoing Laparoscopic Bariatric Surgery. Anesthesiology 2009;110(4):878–84.

94. Zarbock A, Mueller E, Netzer S, et al. Prophylactic nasal continuous positive airway pressure following cardiac surgery protects from postoperative pulmonary complications: a prospective, randomized, controlled trial in 500 patients. Chest 2009;135(5):1252–9.

95. Ferreyra GP, Baussano I, Squadrone V, et al. Continuous positive airway pressure for treatment of respiratory complications after abdominal surgery - A systematic review and meta-analysis. Annals of surgery 2008;247(4):617–26.

96. Jaber S, Delay JM, Chanques G, et al. Outcomes of patients with acute respiratory failure after abdominal surgery treated with noninvasive positive pressure ventilation. Chest 2005;128(4):2688–95.

97. Jaber S, Lescot T, Futier E, et al. Effect of Noninvasive Ventilation on Tracheal Reintubation Among Patients With Hypoxemic Respiratory Failure Following Abdominal Surgery A Randomized Clinical Trial. JAMA, J Am Med Assoc 2016;315(13):1345–53.

98. Squadrone V, Coha M, Cerutti E, et al. Continuous positive airway pressure for treatment of postoperative hypoxemia - A randomized controlled trial. JAMA, J Am Med Assoc 2005;293(5):589–95.

99. Hiramatsu T, Sugiyama M, Kuwabara S, et al. Effectiveness of an outpatient preoperative care bundle in preventing postoperative pneumonia among esophageal cancer patients. Am J Infect Control 2014;42(4):385–8.

100. Mahama G, Vigneswaran L, Silva A, et al. A bundled approach to care: reducing the incidence of postoperative pneumonia in patients undergoing hepatectomy and Whipple procedures. Can J Surg 2021;64(1):E9–13.

101. Caparelli ML, Shikhman A, Jalal A, et al. Prevention of Postoperative Pneumonia in Noncardiac Surgical Patients: A Prospective Study Using the National Surgical Quality Improvement Program Database. Am Surg 2019;85(1):8–14.

102. Cassidy MR, Rosenkranz P, McCabe K, et al. COUGH: reducing postoperative pulmonary complications with a multidisciplinary patient care program. JAMA surgery 2013;148(8):740–5.

Pharmacokinetic and Pharmacodynamic Changes in the Elderly: Impact on Anesthetics

Ettienne Coetzee, MBChB, MMed, FCA (SA)[a],
Anthony Ray Absalom, MBChB, FRCA, MD (UCT)[b],*

KEYWORDS

- Aging • Senescence • Pharmacokinetics • Pharmacodynamics • Frailty
- Physiology

KEY POINTS

- The population demographics in most countries are changing rapidly, causing the number and proportion of elderly patients to increase significantly.
- A growing proportion of the work of anesthesiologists will comprise care of frail elderly patients.
- Age-related physiologic changes result in significant changes in the relationship between drug dose and plasma concentration (pharmacokinetics) and also in the sensitivity of an elderly patient to a given plasma concentration (pharmacodynamics).
- As a result of these changes, the elderly need lower bolus doses and infusion rates of drugs than their younger counterparts for the same clinical effects.
- Even with adjusted doses, the incidence and severity of some adverse effects may be increased.

INTRODUCTION

Anesthesiologists are increasingly being involved in the care of elderly and frail patients because of considerable changes in population demographics, coupled with significant improvements in medical knowledge and technology, and changes in social norms and health policy. Increasingly complex diagnostic and therapeutic techniques have been introduced, and advanced age is no longer seen as a legitimate barrier to surgery and anesthesia.

Whether anesthesiologists are active in the operating theaters, intensive care, or elsewhere, an increasing proportion of their work will involve the administration of

[a] Department of Anaesthesia and Perioperative Medicine, Groote Schuur Hospital, D23, Observatory, Cape Town 7925, Republic of South Africa; [b] Department of Anesthesiology, University of Groningen, University Medical Center Groningen, Post Box 30.001, Groningen 9700 RB, the Netherlands
* Corresponding author.
E-mail address: a.r.absalom@umcg.nl

Anesthesiology Clin 41 (2023) 549–565
https://doi.org/10.1016/j.anclin.2023.02.006
1932-2275/23/© 2023 Elsevier Inc. All rights reserved.

anesthesiology.theclinics.com

sedative, analgesic, and anesthetic drugs to elderly people. This vulnerable population group is very sensitive to the effects of these drugs because of aging-related alterations in pharmacokinetics (PKs)—the relationship between drug dose and achieved plasma concentration—and because of changes in pharmacodynamics (PDs)—the relationship between achieved plasma concentration and clinical effect. This review therefore summarizes the recent literature on PK and PD changes in the elderly.

PHARMACOKINETIC CHANGES IN THE ELDERLY
Physiologic Changes Relevant to Pharmacokinetics

The underlying reasons for, and mechanisms of, senescence, or biological aging, are the subject of intense research. Aging affects not only individual cells but also organs and the whole body. The physiologic changes associated with aging are well-described, with little new published information on this topic. For succinct summaries of the changes most relevant to general and anesthetic pharmacology see the reviews of McLean[1] and Shafer.[2]

In short, aging is associated with changes in body composition and organ function. The function of all organs declines. Although cardiac output is usually only modestly affected, sympathetic tone declines and the ability of the heart to adapt to changes is impaired. Hemodynamic suppression by anesthetic drugs is ascribed to a decrease in peripheral vascular resistance as a result of decreased sympathetic vasoconstrictor nerve activity, more than to a direct vasodilator effect.[3] In addition, systemic vascular compliance increases, which reduces the stressed vascular volume.[4] This reduces left ventricular preload and stroke volume.[5,6] In patients with intact myocardial function, this is usually accompanied by a counterclockwise shift of the Frank–Starling curve to maintain cardiac output,[4] but this compensatory mechanism might be absent in patients with cardiovascular risk factors or disease. Other factors exacerbating hypotensive responses to anesthetic drugs include the use of diuretics and antihypertensives, reduced myocardial and vascular compliance, age-related blunting of beta-adrenergic responses, and the increased prevalence of comorbidities, such as atherosclerosis and diabetes mellitus resulting in autonomic reflex dysfunction.[7]

Renal blood flow, and thus glomerular flow rate, and creatinine clearance decline in parallel with age, which is relevant to drugs that undergo renal clearance. Hepatic mass and blood flow also all decrease with age, causing decreases in clearance by hepatic metabolism of several anesthetic drugs. With regard to body composition, total body water volume decreases,[8] resulting in lower volumes of distribution and therefore higher plasma concentrations of hydrophilic drugs. Muscle mass declines, and partly as a consequence, fat forms a relatively greater proportion of the total body mass. This is important because muscle tissues are considered to be "pharmacokinetically active" as they have a high blood flow, and participate in distribution of most anesthetic drugs, whereas fat tissues have a lower blood flow, but a high capacity to slowly absorb drugs, and in particular fat-soluble drugs. Consequently, volumes of distribution of lipophilic drugs can be similar or even higher in elderly patients compared with younger patients. Aging is also associated with changes in the composition of the blood, with lower concentrations of plasma proteins, including albumin, causing significant changes in the unbound (and therefore active) fraction of highly protein bound drugs.

Most of these changes, with the exception of changes in free fraction of drugs, are reflected in the parameters of drugs for which age-adjusted PK models are available (see below). Almost all of them result in the elderly needing smaller doses to achieve the same plasma concentrations as in younger people, and particularly infusion rates when anesthetic drugs are administered by continuous infusion.

Effects of Aging on Pharmacokinetic Processes

Absorption

In daily anesthetic practice, absorption is relevant when drugs are administered via the oral, rectal, intranasal, buccal, transcutaneous, or inhalational routes. Although aging may not directly influence absorption rates across mucous membranes,[9] other aging-associated physiologic changes can still influence absorption rates. The rates of absorption are influenced by concentration gradients, which depend on delivery rates to the absorption site and rates of removal of drug distal to the absorption site. In the case of inhalational anesthesia, the minute volume of ventilation will have an influence on alveolar delivery and concentrations, and for orally administered drugs, gastric emptying and small and large bowel peristaltic activity may all theoretically influence absorption. Aging is associated with slower gastric emptying rates, which is relevant to drugs that are administered orally but are absorbed from the small bowel. Although paracetamol (acetaminophen) is absorbed by passive diffusion from the small bowel, the time to maximum plasma concentration (Tmax) and maximum plasma concentration (Cmax) after oral administration are not different in elderly patients.[10,11]

Aging-associated reductions in cardiac output and organ perfusion, which are relevant to the removal of drug distal from the absorption site, reduce transmembrane gradients and absorption rates. Other relevant changes that influence absorption include aging-related changes in gastric acidity and also the effects of concomitant medications that may alter gastric acidity or delay gastric and small bowel emptying. For example, a reduction in gastric acidity by proton pump inhibitor use will increase the ionized fraction of aspirin, an acidic drug, thereby reducing gastric absorption.

It is unclear what effect aging-related changes in the nasal mucosa have on intranasal absorption rates. In a study of the safety and tolerability of intranasal dexmedetomidine in elderly patients, noncompartmental PK parameters showed that the mean Tmax was 70 minutes,[12] whereas in a study in younger adults, it was 38 minutes.[13] In an observational study of the use of intranasal midazolam administration in elderly patients with major neurocognitive disorder and care-resistant behavior (mean age 84 years), the time to maximum sedation was 17 minutes.[14] The results of a recent study of the PKs of intranasally administered midazolam in elderly volunteers are not yet available.

Distribution

The PKs of most anesthetic drugs can be explained mathematically by a three-compartment model, which involves two distribution compartments. In the first compartment (central compartment or V1), the volume into which drugs are "immediately" distributed after intravenous administration is relatively unaffected by age. The other two compartments mathematically represent two distribution processes, implying that there are two separate distribution processes with different time constants and capacities.

The first distribution process is rapid distribution into a so-called fast distribution compartment (V2), representing distribution into well-perfused tissues, such as muscles and organs. For many anesthetic drugs, such as propofol, thiopentone, and fentanyl, it is this rapid distribution that limits the duration of the clinical effect. Given the abovementioned changes in muscle mass and organ size and perfusion, rapid distribution is generally slower in elderly patients, meaning that after a bolus dose, plasma concentrations, and eventually also the clinical effect, decline more slowly.

The second distribution process is a slower distribution into a third compartment (V3), representing poorly perfused tissues, such as fat. Although this process is slow, these tissues have a high capacity to absorb drugs, especially lipophilic drugs. Given the body composition changes in the elderly, this process may be similar, or slower, but with a similar or even larger capacity to store drugs, meaning that particularly lipophilic may have a greater tendency to accumulate in the elderly. In noncompartmental PK terms, this will be reflected in a slower elimination half-life.

As a result, the overall volume of distribution V_D (in compartmental kinetics, this is represented by the sum of the compartments) can be increased in the elderly, particularly with lipophilic drugs.

Metabolism

Hepatic blood flow decreases by 10% per decade of life, and hepatic mass also decreases significantly. Most drugs used by anesthesiologists are inactivated by hepatic metabolism. The amount of active drug removed from the blood per unit of time depends on the hepatic blood flow and the hepatic extraction ratio (the fraction of the drug passing through the liver that is removed from the blood stream). Extraction ratios depend on lipid solubility and the activity of the metabolizing enzymes (most commonly from the cytochrome P450 group).[15] For drugs with high extraction ratios, such as propofol and lidocaine, the rate of metabolism strongly depends on hepatic blood flow, and in the elderly, this is the main factor slowing metabolism. For other anesthetic drugs, rates of metabolism will be influenced by reductions in hepatic flow as well as by changes in enzyme activity. Many drugs used by elderly patients, including many anesthetic drugs, are either cytochrome P450 inhibitors or activators.

Metabolic clearance rates exceed hepatic flow rates. The renal metabolism of propofol (extraction ratio 0.6–0.7) accounts for up to one-third of propofol metabolism, and metabolism may also occur in the bowel and lung.[16] Although the age-related changes in renal blood flow, renal mass, and glomerular flow rate are likely to influence renal propofol metabolism, there are a paucity of data to confirm this.

Excretion

Many anesthetic drugs are excreted by the kidney, with either the parent drug being excreted in unchanged form (relevant to smaller hydrophilic drugs that are ionized in plasma, such as rocuronium), or excretion of water-soluble metabolites resulting from hepatic metabolism of the parent (such as morphine 6- and morphine 3-glucuronide, active metabolites of morphine). Drugs can enter the renal tubules by one or more of glomerular filtration, proximal tubule secretion, or distal tubule diffusion.[15] The several ways in which aging can influence the overall excretory capacity of the kidneys have been summarized previously.[17]

Several drugs are excreted changed or unchanged in the bile. Examples include larger molecules such as the aminosteroid muscle relaxants (eg, rocuronium and pancuronium), morphine metabolites, and rifampicin. Modern volatile agents undergo minimal metabolism and are primarily excreted by the lung.

Age-related reductions in organ blood flow and function result in slower excretion of drugs that are excreted by the kidneys, liver, and lungs.

AGE AS A COVARIATE IN PHARMACOKINETIC MODELS FOR ANESTHETIC DRUGS

A few of the older PK models for anesthetic drugs included age as a covariate. A notable exception was the Maitre model for alfentanil which estimated that metabolic clearance decreases linearly with age and used a slower estimate of slow redistribution clearance in patients older than 40 years.[18]

Some more recently published PK models have included age as a covariate. In the Schneider PK model for propofol, the size of V2 decreases linearly with age, resulting in the model estimating slower rates of fast distribution and a lower capacity for fast distribution in elderly patients.[19] Likewise, the Eleveld propofol model also estimates slower fast distribution with advancing age, albeit in a mathematically more complex way.[20] For remifentanil, the Minto model[21,22] adjusts V1 and V2 linearly with age, resulting in decreasing estimates for metabolic, fast distribution and slow distribution clearance with advancing age, consistent with clinical observation that elderly patients require smaller inductions doses, and lower infusion rates than younger patients. The more recently published Eleveld and Kim models for remifentanil also adjust for age. The Eleveld model estimates smaller volumes of all compartments and slow rates of metabolic, fast, and slow distribution clearance,[23] and the Kim model estimates smaller volumes of all compartments and slower metabolic and fast distribution clearance.[24]

The age-related adjustments in these models are all concordant with the known aging-associated changes in the PKs of these drugs. When these models are used for controlling target-controlled infusions (TCI), they will result in older patients receiving one or more of smaller induction bolus sizes and lower maintenance infusion rates for the same target concentrations as in younger patients.

Despite the known aging-related physiologic changes, the PKs of dexmedetomidine do not seem to change appreciably with increasing age.[25] Recently, two new PK models for dexmedetomidine have been published, but none of them adjust the PK parameters in elderly patients.[26,27] These models are also intended to be used as TCI with broad applicability.

The PKs of remimazolam do not seem to be significantly affected by age or organ dysfunction.[28,29]

PHARMACODYNAMIC CHANGES IN THE ELDERLY
Overview of Physiologic Changes Resulting in Differences in Pharmacodynamics in the Elderly

The Reasons for the well-known heightened sensitivity of the elderly to the effects of drugs acting on the central nervous system have not been fully elucidated. Factors thought to increase the sensitivity of older patients include aging-related reductions in cerebral volume and blood flow (which will also slow the onset of clinical effects), cortical thinning, accumulating white matter lesions, altered numbers, and functions of receptors with binding sites for anesthetic drugs (such as gamma aminobutyric acid type A [GABA$_A$], N-methyl-D-aspartate [NMDA], and opioid receptors), declining number and function of neuronal synapses, alterations in autonomic tone and adrenergic receptors, and changes in Ca^{2+} homeostasis.[30,31]

The loss of consciousness coincides with an increase in slow wave power in the electroencephalogram. After the loss of consciousness, the power in the low frequencies reaches a plateau, the height of which correlates with gray matter volume.[32,33] This suggests, but does not prove, that the reduction of cortical volume with aging is part of what increases the sensitivity of elderly patients to the hypnotic drugs.

The loss of consciousness is preceded by and associated with disruption of information transfer and functional connectivity.[34,35] Studies of the relationships among aging, cognitive function, and functional connectivity suggest that aging and cognitive decline (both of which are associated with sensitivity to the anesthetic drugs) are associated with reductions in resting state functional connectivity, but not with changes in cortical volume.[36] Juxtaposing these sets of information suggests that aging-related reductions in functional connectivity are likely responsible for the observation that for a given plasma or effect-site concentration, the elderly show more profound clinical effects than younger patients.

Pharmacodynamic Differences with Commonly Used Drugs in the Elderly

Volatile anesthetics

Meta-analyses consistently show a decreasing log–linear relationship of median alveolar concentration (MAC) with increasing age.[37–39] A recent meta-analysis, which included 1466 patients in the final cohort, found a similar decline in MAC of approximately 6.5% per decade after the age of 1 year.[39] Appropriate adjustment of volatile delivery might facilitate the prevention of known volatile side-effects, such as hypotension, especially in an at-risk, elderly population.

Despite the abovementioned findings, data from clinical practice suggest that clinicians only implement modest reductions, of approximately 3% per decade, in volatile concentrations (**Fig. 1**).[40–42] Only one of the three studies was performed at an institution where the anesthetic machines displayed age-adjusted MAC (aaMAC).[40] Even with correctly displayed aaMAC, clinicians did not sufficiently lower the end-tidal volatile concentration. This alludes to either a lack of awareness, or an unwillingness to use aaMAC, or the presence of other factors that alter their clinical decisions. Although most modern anesthetic machines can calculate and display the aaMAC, different manufacturers use different equations, resulting in calculated aaMAC values differing by up to 23%,[37,43] which might also contribute to a hesitancy for adopting aaMAC, especially in the demanding setting of a busy operating theater.

The use of aaMAC seems to be a safe and robust method to administer age-appropriate volatile concentrations while avoiding accidental awareness under anesthesia.[44,45] There are still contradicting findings in the literature regarding the influence of the use of processed electroencephalographic (pEEG) monitoring in the elderly on perioperative outcomes (such as mortality, postoperative delirium, or cognitive dysfunction).[41,46–53] EEG monitoring could, however, be a useful adjunct, especially in the hands of an anesthetist with basic knowledge on raw EEG patterns associated with anesthesia.[54] The recently updated guideline to the standards of monitoring during anesthesia from the Association of Anaesthetists includes aaMAC as a specific prerequisite during volatile anesthesia.[55]

Propofol

With an aging surgical population and increasing environmental concerns about the volatile anesthetics, it is likely that the use of total intravenous anesthesia (TIVA) in the elderly will increase substantially. Whether performed by a manually controlled infusion or by a TCI pump, propofol's predictable PDs and favorable PKs have

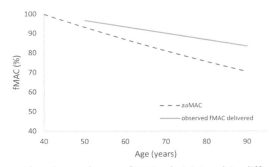

Fig. 1. aaMAC versus the observed mean fMAC administered in different studies. fMAC, fraction of median alveolar concentration required for 50% probability of movement in patients after a standard noxious stimulus; aaMAC, age-adjusted MAC[38]; observed fMAC, the average observed fMAC administered to elderly patients.[40–42]

made it the preferred hypnotic agent during induction of anesthesia and increasingly also during maintenance as part of a TIVA technique.

Current dosing recommendations advise a decreased induction dose size of 1 to 1.5 mg/kg and a maintenance infusion reduction of approximately 50% when compared with younger adults.[56] These lower doses are usually sufficient because of the PKs and PD differences in the elderly. Nonetheless, recent studies found that most anesthesiologists do not adhere to these recommendations during induction of anesthesia, which often leads to excessive depth of anesthesia and clinically relevant cardiovascular impairment.[57–59]

Hypotension

Even without excessive dosing, hypotension can occur in the elderly. For the reasons explained above, elderly patients experience more severe hypotension at equipotent levels of propofol anesthesia, as measured by EEG indices than their younger counterpart.[60] Moreover, the onset of hypotension can also be significantly later than in younger patients, [60,61] which might cause delays or even failure to start supportive interventions. Slower administration rates during induction of anesthesia reduce the overall propofol dose required for the loss of consciousness and lessens the post-induction cardiovascular impairment. [62,63] Infusion rates of 300 mL/h (10 mg every 10 seconds), continued until the loss of consciousness, result in less hypotension and only a modest increase in the induction time (approximately 100 seconds compared with 30–60 seconds), a compromise that seems prudent to preserve hemodynamic stability.

Various coadministration techniques are used to attempt to limit the propofol induction dose and/or attenuate the adrenergic response to laryngoscopy and intubation. Drugs used include benzodiazepines, such as midazolam, and opioids, such as fentanyl, alfentanil, or remifentanil. Although these agents may reduce the propofol induction dose by as much as 50%, they do not always diminish the cardiovascular suppression associated with induction of anesthesia.[64–66] The duration and magnitude of hypotension can occasionally even be increased, in addition to the occurrence of other unwanted effects such as delayed emergence. When coadministration techniques are used for induction of anesthesia, the respective PK profiles of additional anesthetic agents should be carefully considered, along with their potential for additive or even supra-additive PD interaction, before they are administered. There should be a high index of suspicion for peri-induction hypotension.

As mentioned, hypotension can be attenuated by appropriate propofol dosage, slower administration, and titration to clinical effect, following the old adage, "start low, go slow." Judicious intravenous fluid administration, invasive pressure monitoring, and vasopressor administration are other considerations. It is becoming increasingly common for anesthesiologists to start low-dose vasopressor infusions even before induction of anesthesia. Not only the measured blood pressure but also the further reaching effects of vasopressor therapy on cardiac output and oxygen delivery should be taken into account.[67]

Total intravenous anesthesia

During total intravenous anesthesia, propofol is often coadministered with a potent opioid such as remifentanil. Whereas the clinical effects of propofol are mainly mediated by actions at supraspinal levels, the opioids act at supraspinal and spinal levels. This combination capitalizes on the PD interaction between the two drugs to reduce propofol dose requirements to induce and maintain unconsciousness while also promoting immobility which is largely mediated by effects on spinal cord reflexes.[68] The anesthesiologist should bear in mind the effects of aging on the PK and PD of remifentanil, so avoid excessive doses of remifentanil (which could in turn exacerbate hypotension).

Given the sensitivity of the elderly to propofol, an important consideration is the use of pEEG monitoring as a measure of clinical effect. Clinical experience shows that in the majority of elderly patients, pEEG or even raw EEG waveform monitoring (to detect burst suppression) will reveal that anesthetic depth is excessive and the infusion rates can be reduced.

In countries where the technology is available,[69,70] the use of TCI pumps for propofol and remifentanil administration may have added value, particularly now that there are pharmacokinetic and pharmacodynamic (PKPD) models for these drugs that adjust the necessary infusion rates for age. TCI pumps are computer-controlled infusion pumps that calculate and implement the required infusion rates to achieve and maintain the user-defined target plasma or effect-site concentration. The algorithms in the pumps use PKPD models, along with the patient characteristics such as age, weight, height, and sex to calculate and adjust the infusion rates over time, thereby maintaining stable plasma concentrations with reduced cognitive workload for the anesthesiologist and with an excellent safety record.[71]

The propofol PKPD model developed by Eleveld and colleagues [20] has recently been prospectively validated [72] and has already been incorporated in some TCI pumps available in Europe. This model incorporates a set of PD parameters that can be used to estimate age-dependent effects of any given dose and plasma concentration on the bispectral index (BIS). It can also be used in the reverse to determine the effect-site concentration (and hence also the infusion rates) necessary for a given desired BIS value. The PD aspects of the model were developed from five studies containing patients characteristics, propofol infusion rates, and BIS values. In this data set, the baseline BIS was 94. The Ce_{50} was therefore the effect-site concentration required for a BIS of 47—a reasonable target during general anesthesia—and the Ce_{10} the concentration required for a BIS of 84, a reasonable goal during sedation. Consistent with prior knowledge, age has a strong effect on these and all values. **Fig. 2** shows the influence of age on the effect-site concentrations necessary for a BIS of 50 as estimated by the Eleveld model.

Remifentanil

Opioids are used for their potent analgesic effects. In clinically used doses, they have little effect on the EEG, but at concentrations much higher than those needed for analgesia they also produce dose-dependent, predictable changes in the EEG. [73] During the development of the Minto model for remifentanil, EEG signals were recorded to objectively measure cortical drug effect and quantify the age-related changes in the sensitivity to the drug.[21,22] **Fig. 3** illustrates the influence of age on the Ce_{50} of remifentanil for EEG effects.

The time course of the analgesic effects of remifentanil has recently been shown to be much slower than that for the EEG effects and also therefore the predictions of the Minto model.[74] Nonetheless, the influence of age on the plasma and effect-site remifentanil concentrations required for analgesia is likely to be of a similar magnitude.

The data from Minto and colleagues suggest that the combined PK and PD differences in elderly patients reduce their dose requirements to as little as *one-third* of that required in young patients.[21] In addition, they found an age-dependent increase in the time to maximum drug effect. The time to peak drug effect is nearly doubled in elderly patients, occurring more than 2 minutes after a bolus dose is given. The increased sensitivity and slower onset of action should prompt clinicians to either reduce the

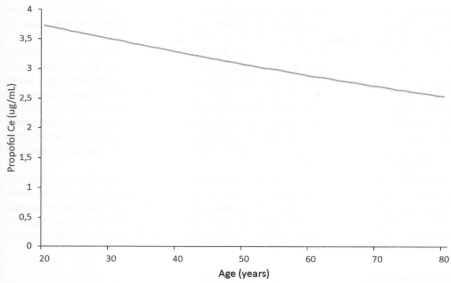

Fig. 2. Influence of age on the propofol effect-site concentration required for a BIS of 50, as estimated by the Eleveld model. (*Data from* Eleveld DJ, Colin P, Absalom AR, Struys M. Pharmacokinetic-pharmacodynamic model for propofol for broad application in anaesthesia and sedation. Br J Anaesth. May 2018;120(5):942-959. https://doi.org/10.1016/j.bja.2018.01.018.)

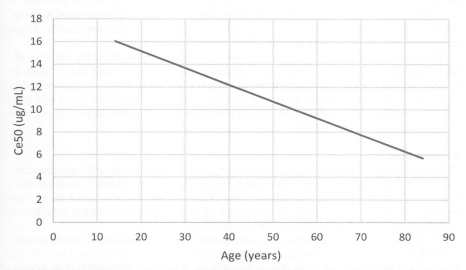

Fig. 3. Influence of age on the Ce_{50} of remifentanil to decrease the electroencephalogram spectral edge frequency.[21] Ce_{50}: Effect-site concentration of remifentanil that produces 50% of the maximal decrease in spectral edge frequency on the electroencephalogram. (*Data from* Minto CF, Schnider TW, Egan TD, et al. Influence of age and gender on the pharmacokinetics and pharmacodynamics of remifentanil. I. Model development. Anesthesiology. 1997;86(1):10-23.)

bolus dose by at least 50%, followed by similar reductions in the maintenance dose with adequate allowance for the increased time to effect, before titrating the dose upwards. Alternatively, the bolus dose can be omitted.

The synergistic PD interaction between remifentanil and other hypnotics, such as volatiles and propofol, has also been well described[68,75–79] and should always be kept in mind when combinations involving remifentanil are used. A recent study found that a remifentanil infusion of 0.125 μg/kg/min, started 3 minutes before induction of anesthesia, reduced the induction dose of propofol by approximately 20%.[65] Taken together these data suggest that in the elderly, lower doses, infusion rates, and target concentrations of remifentanil should be used in the elderly and that the infusion rates or target concentrations should only be increased after a longer period of time has passed than in younger patients.

In-depth PKPD interaction models, specifically aimed at the elderly, are not currently available. This interaction should, however, be carefully considered when combining remifentanil with other anesthetic agents that could cause both wanted and unwanted effects. Remifentanil has been used successfully in elderly patients with significant cardiovascular disease, with fewer side-effects when administered by TCI.[80,81]

Dexmedetomidine

Dexmedetomidine is a highly selective α_2-adrenoreceptor agonist, with sedative and analgesic properties that produce sedation from which patients are easily rousable from, with minimal respiratory suppressive effects, [82] properties that make it an appealing option for monitored anesthetic care or procedural sedation. Recent literature suggests that using perioperative dexmedetomidine might also reduce postoperative delirium, a complication that is common in the elderly and associated with significant morbidity.[83–85] When used for procedural sedation in elderly patients, it has been shown to be associated with fewer periprocedural complications, such as hypotension and respiratory adverse events, and improved sedation quality, when compared with propofol, remifentanil, or benzodiazepines.[86–88]

Elderly patients seem to be more sensitive than younger patients to the sedative effects, and hypotension occurred more frequently when a loading dose of 0.7 μg/kg or greater were administered. Current literature does not recommend an age-adjusted dose but caution is warranted when the drug is used in frail patients or those with cardiovascular disease, especially if it is used in conjunction with other agents that could enhance cardiovascular suppression.

Remimazolam

Remimazolam is an ultra-short-acting benzodiazepine that was recently approved for use as a general anesthetic in Japan and South Korea, and for procedural sedation in China, Europe, South Korea, and the United States.[28] Large-scale data sets are still lacking, but recent studies suggest that remimazolam may have a future in procedural sedation and general anesthesia in elderly patients.[89–92]

Elderly patients seem to have increased sensitivity to remimazolam. Current recommendations support administration of a bolus dose of 2.5 to 5 mg over 1 minute for induction of sedation. For induction of anesthesia, the recommendation is to administer an infusion at a rate of 6 mg/kg/h in healthy adults and significantly lower rates in the elderly. The median effective total dose for induction of anesthesia was recently reported to be 0.09 mg/kg in patients of 65 years and approximately 0.06 mg/kg in patients over 75 years.[93] Elderly patients are also at increased risk for delayed emergence and extubation.[94] Larger, patient-specific studies are warranted to establish a "general purpose" PKPD model, with broad spectrum application for both procedural sedation and general anesthesia.

SUMMARY

With the aging population, anesthesiologists and intensivists will increasingly be required to care for frail elderly patients. A detailed knowledge of the influence of age on the PKs and dynamics of the anesthetic drugs is required for optimal safety and attenuation of adverse effects. For most of the anesthetic drugs, the elderly needs lower doses to achieve the same plasma concentrations as in younger patients, and at any given plasma and effect-site concentration, elderly patients will have more profound clinical effects. In the elderly in particular, caution is required, with close monitoring of clinical effects and active titration of dose administration to achieve the desired level of effect, ideally following the "start low, go slow" principle.

CLINICS CARE POINTS

- Senescence leads to changes in the pharmacokinetics and pharmacodynamics of anesthetic drugs, leading to a reduction in the dosage required for a given effect, increasing the likelihood of adverse effects and ultimately leading to a narrower therapeutic window.

- Consider the impact of end-organ function on drug pharmacokinetics when selecting anesthetic drugs in elderly patients.

- Appropriate age-adjusted minimum alveolar concentrations should be used when volatile anesthesia is administered.

- Post-induction hypotension can be attenuated by administering a smaller bolus dose of hypnotic at a slower rate and taking into account the expected delay in onset of clinical effect before administration of an additional bolus.

- When combinations of a hypnotic and opioid are administered, the strong pharmacodynamic synergism between these categories of drugs will reduce the amount of hypnotic needed.

- Where available, target-controlled infusion systems should be used during total intravenous anesthesia.

- When administering drugs to the elderly using target-controlled infusion technology, it is advisable to use a pharmacokinetic model that incorporates *age as a covariate*, such as the Eleveld and Schnider models for propofol and the Minto and Kim models for remifentanil.

- Evidence suggests that monitoring of the perioperative electroencephalogram might aid in individualizing hypnotic induction and maintenance doses.

DISCLOSURE

E. Coetzee has no disclosures to declare. A.R. Absalom is a trustee of the BJA charity. His department has been reimbursed for sponsor-initiated phase I research by The Medicines Company and Rigel Inc. His department has been reimbursed for consultancy advice to Philips, Johnson and Johnson (Janssen Pharma), Ever Pharma, PAION, The Medicines Company, and Terumo.

FUNDING

The work was funded by internal departmental resources.

REFERENCES

1. McLean AJ, Le Couteur DG. Aging biology and geriatric clinical pharmacology. Pharmacol Rev 2004;56(2):163–84.
2. Shafer SL. The pharmacology of anesthetic drugs in elderly patients. Anesthesiol Clin North Am 2000;18(1):1–29.
3. Robinson BJ, Ebert TJ, O'Brien TJ, et al. Mechanisms whereby propofol mediates peripheral vasodilation in humans. Sympathoinhibition or direct vascular relaxation? Anesthesiology 1997;86(1):64–72.
4. de Wit F, van Vliet AL, de Wilde RB, et al. The effect of propofol on haemodynamics: cardiac output, venous return, mean systemic filling pressure, and vascular resistances. Br J Anaesth 2016;116(6):784–9.
5. Hammaren E, Hynynen M. Haemodynamic effects of propofol infusion for sedation after coronary artery surgery. Br J Anaesth 1995;75(1):47–50.
6. Soleimani A, Heidari N, Habibi MR, et al. Comparing Hemodynamic Responses to Diazepam, Propofol and Etomidate During Anesthesia Induction in Patients with Left Ventricular Dysfunction Undergoing Coronary Artery Bypass Graft Surgery: a Double-blind, Randomized Clinical Trial. Med Arch 2017;71(3):198–203.
7. Priebe HJ. The aged cardiovascular risk patient. Br J Anaesth 2000;85(5): 763–78.
8. Beaufrere B, Morio B. Fat and protein redistribution with aging: metabolic considerations. Eur J Clin Nutr 2000;54(Suppl 3):S48–53.
9. Kharasch ED, Hoffer C, Whittington D. Influence of age on the pharmacokinetics and pharmacodynamics of oral transmucosal fentanyl citrate. Anesthesiology 2004;101(3):738–43.
10. Raffa RB, Pergolizzi JV Jr, Taylor R Jr, et al. Acetaminophen (paracetamol) oral absorption and clinical influences. Pain Pract 2014;14(7):668–77.
11. Mian P, Allegaert K, Spriet I, et al. Paracetamol in Older People: Towards Evidence-Based Dosing? Drugs Aging 2018;35(7):603–24.
12. Barends CRM, Driesens MK, Struys M, et al. Intranasal dexmedetomidine in elderly subjects with or without beta blockade: a randomised double-blind single-ascending-dose cohort study. Br J Anaesth 2020. https://doi.org/10.1016/j.bja.2019.12.025.
13. Iirola T, Vilo S, Manner T, et al. Bioavailability of dexmedetomidine after intranasal administration. Eur J Clin Pharmacol 2011;67(8):825–31.
14. Barends CRM, Absalom AR, Visser A. Intranasal midazolam for the sedation of geriatric patients with care-resistant behaviour during essential dental treatment: An observational study. Gerodontology 2022;39(2):161–9.
15. Peck T, Harris B. Pharmacology for anaesthesia and intensive care. 5 edition. Cambridge University Press; 2021.
16. Sahinovic MM, Struys M, Absalom AR. Clinical Pharmacokinetics and Pharmacodynamics of Propofol. Clin Pharmacokinet 2018;57(12):1539–58.
17. Akhtar S. Pharmacological considerations in the elderly. Curr Opin Anaesthesiol 2018;31(1):11–8.
18. Maitre PO, Vozeh S, Heykants J, et al. Population pharmacokinetics of alfentanil: the average dose- plasma concentration relationship and interindividual variability in patients. Anesthesiology 1987;66:3–12.
19. Schnider TW, Minto CF, Gambus PL, et al. The influence of method of administration and covariates on the pharmacokinetics of propofol in adult volunteers. Anesthesiology 1998;88(5):1170–82.

20. Eleveld DJ, Colin P, Absalom AR, et al. Pharmacokinetic-pharmacodynamic model for propofol for broad application in anaesthesia and sedation. Br J Anaesth 2018;120(5):942–59.

21. Minto CF, Schnider TW, Egan TD, et al. Influence of age and gender on the pharmacokinetics and pharmacodynamics of remifentanil. I. Model development. Anesthesiology 1997;86(1):10–23.

22. Minto CF, Schnider TW, Shafer SL. Pharmacokinetics and pharmacodynamics of remifentanil. II. Model application. Anesthesiology 1997;86(1):24–33.

23. Eleveld DJ, Proost JH, Vereecke H, et al. An Allometric Model of Remifentanil Pharmacokinetics and Pharmacodynamics. Anesthesiology 2017;126(6): 1005–18.

24. Kim TK, Obara S, Egan TD, et al. Disposition of Remifentanil in Obesity: A New Pharmacokinetic Model Incorporating the Influence of Body Mass. Anesthesiology 2017;126(6):1019–32.

25. Weerink MAS, Struys M, Hannivoort LN, et al. Clinical Pharmacokinetics and Pharmacodynamics of Dexmedetomidine. Clin Pharmacokinet 2017;56(8): 893–913.

26. Morse JD, Cortinez LI, Anderson BJ. A Universal Pharmacokinetic Model for Dexmedetomidine in Children and Adults. J Clin Med 2020;9(11). https://doi.org/10. 3390/jcm9113480.

27. Hannivoort LN, Eleveld DJ, Proost JH, et al. Development of an Optimized Pharmacokinetic Model of Dexmedetomidine Using Target-controlled Infusion in Healthy Volunteers. Anesthesiology 2015;123(2):357–67.

28. Kim KM. Remimazolam: pharmacological characteristics and clinical applications in anesthesiology. Anesth Pain Med (Seoul) 2022;17(1):1–11.

29. Masui K, Stohr T, Pesic M, et al. A population pharmacokinetic model of remimazolam for general anesthesia and consideration of remimazolam dose in clinical practice. J Anesth 2022;36(4):493–505.

30. Kruijt Spanjer MR, Bakker NA, Absalom AR. Pharmacology in the elderly and newer anaesthesia drugs. Best Pract Res Clin Anaesthesiol 2011;25(3):355–65.

31. Vuyk J. Pharmacodynamics in the elderly. Best Pract Res Clin Anaesthesiol 2003; 17(2):207–18.

32. Ni Mhuircheartaigh R, Warnaby C, Rogers R, et al. Slow-wave activity saturation and thalamocortical isolation during propofol anesthesia in humans. Sci translational Med 2013;5(208). 208ra148.

33. Warnaby CE, Sleigh JW, Hight D, et al. Investigation of Slow-wave Activity Saturation during Surgical Anesthesia Reveals a Signature of Neural Inertia in Humans. Anesthesiology 2017;127(4):645–57.

34. Pullon RM, Yan L, Sleigh JW, et al. Granger Causality of the Electroencephalogram Reveals Abrupt Global Loss of Cortical Information Flow during Propofol-induced Loss of Responsiveness. Anesthesiology 2020;133(4):774–86.

35. Pullon RM, Warnaby CE, Sleigh JW. Propofol-induced Unresponsiveness Is Associated with a Brain Network Phase Transition. Anesthesiology 2022;136(3): 420–33.

36. Schulz M, Mayer C, Schlemm E, et al. Association of Age and Structural Brain Changes With Functional Connectivity and Executive Function in a Middle-Aged to Older Population-Based Cohort. Front Aging Neurosci 2022;14:782738.

37. Mapleson WW. Effect of age on MAC in humans: a meta-analysis. Br J Anaesth 1996;76(2):179–85.

38. Eger EI 2nd. Age, minimum alveolar anesthetic concentration, and minimum alveolar anesthetic concentration-awake. Anesth Analg 2001;93(4):947–53.

39. Cooter M, Ni K, Thomas J, et al. Age-dependent decrease in minimum alveolar concentration of inhaled anaesthetics: a systematic search of published studies and meta-regression analysis. Br J Anaesth 2020;124(1):e4–7.

40. Hight D, Schanderhazi C, Huber M, et al. Age, minimum alveolar concentration and choice of depth of sedation monitor: examining the paradox of age when using the Narcotrend monitor: A secondary analysis of an observational study. Eur J Anaesthesiol 2022;39(4):305–14.

41. Ni K, Cooter M, Gupta DK, et al. Paradox of age: older patients receive higher age-adjusted minimum alveolar concentration fractions of volatile anaesthetics yet display higher bispectral index values. Br J Anaesth 2019;123(3):288–97.

42. Van Cleve WC, Nair BG, Rooke GA. Associations Between Age and Dosing of Volatile Anesthetics in 2 Academic Hospitals. Anesth Analg 2015;121(3):645–51.

43. Sato N, Terada T, Ochiai R. MAC value of desflurane may vary for different machines. J Anesth 2016;30(1):183.

44. Avidan MS, Mashour GA. Prevention of intraoperative awareness with explicit recall: making sense of the evidence. Anesthesiology 2013;118(2):449–56.

45. Aranake A, Mashour GA, Avidan MS. Minimum alveolar concentration: ongoing relevance and clinical utility. Anaesthesia 2013;68(5):512–22.

46. Short TG, Campbell D, Frampton C, et al. Anaesthetic depth and complications after major surgery: an international, randomised controlled trial. Lancet 2019; 394(10212):1907–14.

47. Wildes TS, Mickle AM, Ben Abdallah A, et al. Effect of Electroencephalography-Guided Anesthetic Administration on Postoperative Delirium Among Older Adults Undergoing Major Surgery: The ENGAGES Randomized Clinical Trial. JAMA 2019;321(5):473–83.

48. Miao M, Xu Y, Sun M, et al. BIS index monitoring and perioperative neurocognitive disorders in older adults: a systematic review and meta-analysis. Aging Clin Exp Res 2020;32(12):2449–58.

49. Evered LA, Chan MTV, Han R, et al. Anaesthetic depth and delirium after major surgery: a randomised clinical trial. Br J Anaesth 2021;127(5):704–12.

50. Ajayan N, Hrishi AP. How balanced is the BALANCED delirium trial? Comment on Br J Anaesth 2021; 127: 704-12. Br J Anaesth 2022;128(4):e274–5.

51. Chew WZ, Teoh WY, Sivanesan N, et al. Bispectral Index (BIS) Monitoring and Postoperative Delirium in Elderly Patients Undergoing Surgery: A Systematic Review and Meta-Analysis With Trial Sequential Analysis. J Cardiothorac Vasc Anesth 2022. https://doi.org/10.1053/j.jvca.2022.07.004.

52. Sumner M, Deng C, Evered L, et al. Processed electroencephalography-guided general anaesthesia to reduce postoperative delirium: a systematic review and meta-analysis. Br J Anaesth 2022;16. https://doi.org/10.1016/j.bja.2022.01.006.

53. Whitlock EL, Gross ER, King CR, et al. Anaesthetic depth and delirium: a challenging balancing act. Br J Anaesth 2021;127(5):667–71.

54. Barnard JP, Bennett C, Voss LJ, et al. Can anaesthetists be taught to interpret the effects of general anaesthesia on the electroencephalogram? Comparison of performance with the BIS and spectral entropy. Br J Anaesth 2007;99(4):532–7.

55. Klein AA, Meek T, Allcock E, et al. Recommendations for standards of monitoring during anaesthesia and recovery 2021: Guideline from the Association of Anaesthetists. Anaesthesia 2021;76(9):1212–23.

56. Kabi F. DIPRIVAN (Propofol) injectable emulsion, USP. . FDA.. Available at: https://www.accessdata.fda.gov/drugsatfda_docs/label/2017/019627s066lbl. pdf. Accessed 30 October 2022.

57. Akhtar S, Heng J, Dai F, et al. A Retrospective Observational Study of Anesthetic Induction Dosing Practices in Female Elderly Surgical Patients: Are We Overdosing Older Patients? Drugs Aging 2016;33(10):737–46.
58. Akhtar S, Liu J, Heng J, et al. Does intravenous induction dosing among patients undergoing gastrointestinal surgical procedures follow current recommendations: a study of contemporary practice. J Clin Anesth 2016;33:208–15.
59. Phillips AT, Deiner S, Mo Lin H, et al. Propofol Use in the Elderly Population: Prevalence of Overdose and Association With 30-Day Mortality. Clin Ther 2015;37(12): 2676–85.
60. Kazama T, Ikeda K, Morita K, et al. Comparison of the effect-site k(eO)s of propofol for blood pressure and EEG bispectral index in elderly and younger patients. Anesthesiology 1999;90(6):1517–27.
61. Su H, Eleveld DJ, Struys M, et al. Mechanism-based pharmacodynamic model for propofol haemodynamic effects in healthy volunteers. Br J Anaesth 2022; 128(5):806–16.
62. Peacock JE, Lewis RP, Reilly CS, et al. Effect of different rates of infusion of propofol for induction of anaesthesia in elderly patients. Br J Anaesth 1990;65(3): 346–52.
63. Kaul TK, Gautam P, Narula N, et al. Effects of different rates of infusion of 1% and 2% propofol for induction of anaesthesia in elderly patients. Indian J Anaesth 2002;46(6):460–4.
64. Cressey DM, Claydon P, Bhaskaran NC, et al. Effect of midazolam pretreatment on induction dose requirements of propofol in combination with fentanyl in younger and older adults. Anaesthesia 2001;56(2):108–13.
65. You AH, Kim JY, Kim DH, et al. Effect of remifentanil and midazolam on ED95 of propofol for loss of consciousness in elderly patients: A randomized, clinical trial. Medicine (Baltimore) 2019;98(16):e15132.
66. Billard V, Moulla F, Bourgain JL, et al. Hemodynamic response to induction and intubation. Propofol/fentanyl Interaction *Anesthesiology* 1994;81(6):1384–93.
67. Ho AM, Mizubuti GB. Co-induction with a vasopressor "chaser" to mitigate propofol-induced hypotension when intubating critically ill/frail patients-A questionable practice. J Crit Care 2019;54:256–60.
68. Struys MM, Vereecke H, Moerman A, et al. Ability of the bispectral index, autoregressive modelling with exogenous input-derived auditory evoked potentials, and predicted propofol concentrations to measure patient responsiveness during anesthesia with propofol and remifentanil. Anesthesiology 2003;99(4):802–12.
69. Absalom AR, Glen JB, Zwart GJC, et al. Target-Controlled Infusion: A Mature Technology. Anesth Analg 2016;122(1):70–8.
70. Struys MM, De Smet T, Glen JI, et al. The History of Target-Controlled Infusion. Anesth Analg 2016;122(1):56–69.
71. Schnider TW, Minto CF, Struys MM, et al. The Safety of Target-Controlled Infusions. Anesth Analg 2016;122(1):79–85.
72. Vellinga R, Hannivoort LN, Introna M, et al. Prospective clinical validation of the Eleveld propofol pharmacokinetic-pharmacodynamic model in general anaesthesia. *Br J Anaesth* Feb 2021;126(2):386–94.
73. Scott JC, Cooke JE, Stanski DR. Electroencephalographic quantitation of opioid effect: comparative pharmacodynamics of fentanyl and sufentanil. Anesthesiology 1991;74:34–42.
74. Abad-Torrent A, Martinez-Vazquez P, Somma J, et al. Remifentanil pharmacodynamics during conscious sedation using algometry: a more clinically relevant

pharmacodynamical model. Br J Anaesth 2022. https://doi.org/10.1016/j.bja.2022.08.026.

75. Nieuwenhuijs DJ, Olofsen E, Romberg RR, et al. Response surface modeling of remifentanil-propofol interaction on cardiorespiratory control and bispectral index. Anesthesiology 2003;98(2):312–22.

76. Kern SE, Xie G, White JL, et al. A response surface analysis of propofol-remifentanil pharmacodynamic interaction in volunteers. Anesthesiology 2004; 100(6):1373–81.

77. Bouillon TW, Bruhn J, Radulescu L, et al. Pharmacodynamic interaction between propofol and remifentanil regarding hypnosis, tolerance of laryngoscopy, bispectral index, and electroencephalographic approximate entropy. Anesthesiology 2004;100(6):1353–72.

78. Johnson KB, Syroid ND, Gupta DK, et al. An evaluation of remifentanil propofol response surfaces for loss of responsiveness, loss of response to surrogates of painful stimuli and laryngoscopy in patients undergoing elective surgery. AnesthAnalg 2008;106(2):471–9.

79. Hannivoort LN, Vereecke HE, Proost JH, et al. Probability to tolerate laryngoscopy and noxious stimulation response index as general indicators of the anaesthetic potency of sevoflurane, propofol, and remifentanil. Br J Anaesth 2016;116(5): 624–31 [doi].

80. De Castro V, Godet G, Mencia G, et al. Target-controlled infusion for remifentanil in vascular patients improves hemodynamics and decreases remifentanil requirement. Anesth Analgesia 2003;96(1):33–8, table of contents.

81. Yamamoto M, Meguro K, Mouillet G, et al. Effect of local anesthetic management with conscious sedation in patients undergoing transcatheter aortic valve implantation. Am J Cardiol 2013;111(1):94–9.

82. Hall JE, Uhrich TD, Barney JA, et al. Sedative, amnestic, and analgesic properties of small-dose dexmedetomidine infusions. Anesth Analgesia 2000;90(3): 699–705.

83. van Norden J, Spies CD, Borchers F, et al. The effect of peri-operative dexmedetomidine on the incidence of postoperative delirium in cardiac and non-cardiac surgical patients: a randomised, double-blind placebo-controlled trial. Anaesthesia 2021;76(10):1342–51.

84. Uusalo P, Seppanen SM, Jarvisalo MJ. Feasibility of Intranasal Dexmedetomidine in Treatment of Postoperative Restlessness, Agitation, and Pain in Geriatric Orthopedic Patients. Drugs Aging 2021;38(5):441–50.

85. Qin C, Jiang Y, Lin C, et al. Perioperative dexmedetomidine administration to prevent delirium in adults after non-cardiac surgery: A systematic review and meta-analysis. J Clin Anesth 2021;73:110308.

86. Mei B, Meng G, Xu G, et al. Intraoperative Sedation With Dexmedetomidine is Superior to Propofol for Elderly Patients Undergoing Hip Arthroplasty: A Prospective Randomized Controlled Study. Clin J Pain 2018;34(9):811–7.

87. Silva JM, Katayama HT, Nogueira FAM, et al. Comparison of dexmedetomidine and benzodiazepine for intraoperative sedation in elderly patients: a randomized clinical trial. Reg Anesth Pain Med 2019;44(3):319–24.

88. Kaya C, Celebi NO, Debbag S, et al. Comparison of dexmedetomidine and remifentanil infusion in geriatric patients undergoing outpatient cataract surgery: a prospective, randomized, and blinded study. Med Gas Res 2022;12(4):146–52.

89. Nakanishi T, Sento Y, Kamimura Y, et al. Remimazolam for induction of anesthesia in elderly patients with severe aortic stenosis: a prospective, observational pilot study. BMC Anesthesiol 2021;21(1):306.

90. Nakayama J, Ogihara T, Yajima R, et al. Anesthetic management of super-elderly patients with remimazolam: a report of two cases. JA Clin Rep 2021;7(1):71.
91. Guo J, Qian Y, Zhang X, et al. Remimazolam tosilate compared with propofol for gastrointestinal endoscopy in elderly patients: a prospective, randomized and controlled study. BMC Anesthesiol 2022;22(1):180.
92. Tan Y, Ouyang W, Tang Y, et al. Effect of remimazolam tosilate on early cognitive function in elderly patients undergoing upper gastrointestinal endoscopy. J Gastroenterol Hepatol 2022;37(3):576–83.
93. Liu M, Sun Y, Zhou L, et al. The Median Effective Dose and Bispectral Index of Remimazolam Tosilate for Anesthesia Induction in Elderly Patients: An Up-and-Down Sequential Allocation Trial. Clin Interv Aging 2022;17:837–43.
94. Shimamoto Y, Sanuki M, Kurita S, et al. Factors affecting prolonged time to extubation in patients given remimazolam. PLoS One 2022;17(5):e0268568.

Update on Perioperative Delirium

Katie J. Schenning, MD, MPH, MCR[a],*, Elizabeth Mahanna-Gabrielli, MD[b],
Stacie G. Deiner, MD[c]

KEYWORDS

- Delirium • Frailty • Cognitive impairment • Anesthesia • Geriatric

KEY POINTS

- Risk factors for frailty are similar to risk factors for postoperative delirium (POD).
- Patients identified as frail could be referred for a preoperative comprehensive geriatric assessment and geriatricians could contribute to postoperative management with multidisciplinary teams executing evidence-based delirium prevention bundles.
- POD has been found to be associated with worse functional recovery in older surgical patients.
- After decades of observational studies, randomized trials, meta-analyses, and systematic reviews, the evidence has never been strong enough to support the choice of regional over general anesthesia for older surgical patients to prevent POD.
- Patients with mild cognitive impairment who have an episode of delirium have worse cognitive decline after surgery compared with patients with mild cognitive impairment who do not have an episode of delirium.

INTRODUCTION

Postoperative delirium (POD) is currently recognized as the most common complication in older surgical patients. Although delirium is common, it is not part of the normal physiology of aging. Although it is an unwanted postoperative outcome, it is also a symptom of an aging brain and a cause of other downstream outcomes. Delirium research has rapidly increased in the past 25 years. This update on perioperative delirium highlights 3 important areas of rapid development. These areas include the relationship between delirium and frailty, the comparison of different types of anesthesia on incident POD, and an improved description of the long-term cognitive consequences of POD.

---

[a] Department of Anesthesiology & Perioperative Medicine, Oregon Health & Science University, 3181 Southwest Sam Jackson Park Road L459, Portland, OR 97239, USA; [b] Department of Anesthesiology, Perioperative Medicine and Pain Management, University of Miami Miller School of Medicine, 2000 S Bayshore Drive Apartment 51, Miami, FL 33133, USA; [c] Department of Anesthesiology, Dartmouth Hitchcock Medical Center, Lebanon, NH, USA
* Corresponding author.
E-mail address: malcore@ohsu.edu

Anesthesiology Clin 41 (2023) 567–581
https://doi.org/10.1016/j.anclin.2023.02.007
1932-2275/23/© 2023 Elsevier Inc. All rights reserved.

FRAILTY AND COGNITIVE IMPAIRMENT

The concept of frailty has been present throughout the history of medicine but only during the past 25 years has frailty come to be precisely defined and measured. Frailty describes the medical condition in which a person is vulnerable to stressors with little resilience or the ability to fully recover due to the decline in function across multiple organ systems.[1] It is accompanied by physical weakness and often by cognitive impairment. Cognitive impairment and frailty frequently coexist, and one is a risk factor for the other. Cognitive frailty is defined as physical frailty accompanied by cognitive impairment but without dementia and was first proposed by the International Academy of Nutrition and Aging and the International Association of Gerontology and Geriatrics in 2013.[2,3] Expanding frailty to a multidimensional syndrome incorporates the vulnerability of older adults associated with cognitive impairment.[2,4] Cognitive frailty describes patients with cognitive vulnerability and reduced resilience and represents cognitive impairment caused by physical conditions and possibly an antecedent to neurodegenerative disease.[2] Physical and cognitive frailty have been associated with decline and dysfunction in the frontal cognitive domains, such as executive function and attention.[2,5]

FRAILTY AND AGING

Although the prevalence of frailty and cognitive frailty increase with age, frailty differs from healthy aging. Healthy aging is accompanied by physiologic changes but these changes do not lead to the severe depletion of reserve and vulnerability even to small stressors.[1] Frailty is present in anywhere from 11% to 59% of community-dwelling adults.[6] It has increased prevalence among people with end-stage renal disease and malignancies.[6] Frailty is increased in women, people with lower socioeconomic status, and in ethnic and racial minorities.[6] Specifically, cognitive frailty is present in 10.7% to 22.0% of patients and 1.0% to 4.4% in community-dwelling adults.[7]

POSTOPERATIVE DELIRIUM AND FRAILTY

Because many of the risk factors for frailty are similar to risk factors for POD, frailty has been investigated as a risk factor for delirium. A recent meta-analysis included studies investigating a relationship between preoperative frailty and POD in patients aged at least 65 years, undergoing elective, nonemergent inpatient surgery.[8] Nine studies involving both cardiac (n = 6) and noncardiac surgery (n = 3) were included in the analysis. The meta-analysis included 1008 subjects with a mean age of 74 years of whom 42% were women. Preoperative frailty was present in 18% to 56% of subjects. Overall, the association of POD in frail versus nonfrail patients was significant (odds ratio [OR] 2.14; 95% confidence interval (CI) of 1.43–3.19).[8] A subsequent meta-analysis included retrospective studies of patients who underwent elective and emergency surgery, and all adult patients regardless of age but did not include studies without multivariate analysis.[9] A total of 15 studies and 3250 subjects were analyzed. Preoperative frailty was identified in 27.1% of subjects and was significantly associated with POD compared with nonfrail patients (OR 3.23; 95% CI: 2.56 to 4.07).[9] The authors found that the association between frailty and POD remained significant in multiple subgroup analyses of age, elective or emergency surgery, cardiac or noncardiac surgery, country of the study, instruments used for identification of frailty or POD, or quality score of the study.[9]

Similarly, a strong association between frailty and in-hospital delirium in nonsurgical patients has been shown. A recent meta-analysis found that frail medical patients had an OR of 3.61 (95% CI 3.61–7.89) for delirium, and frail patients with emergency or critical illness had an OR of 6.66 (95% CI 1.41–31.47) for delirium.[10]

FRAILTY SCALES AND INSTRUMENTS

Frailty can be screened and diagnosed by various tools and instruments. There are 2 main approaches to determining frailty: assessing for a frailty phenotype and assessing for accumulation of medical diseases and deficits. The frailty phenotype first proposed by Fried and Walston comprises 5 components that synergistically cause deterioration: weakness, slowness, fatigue, low activity, and weight loss.[11] The cumulation of medical diseases and deficits approach developed at a similar time and is determined by a count of the number of diseases and medical conditions across all organ systems.[12] Some of the most common phenotype instruments are the fatigue, resistance, ambulation, illness, loss of weight (FRAIL) scale, the Clinical Frailty Scale, the Frailty Phenotype, Gait Speed, and the Gérontopôle Frailty Screening Tool.[11,13–16] The Frailty Phenotype, Gait Speed, and Gérontopôle Frailty Screening Tool all require in-person assessments given the need for the objective measurement of grip strength and gait speed. Although having an objective measurement of strength and resistance has advantages, many preoperative clinics perform patient assessments over the phone limiting the ability to use these types of instruments. Similarly, the Clinical Frailty Scale requires a comprehensive assessment by a provider and is not meant to be performed over the phone.

Alternatively, the FRAIL scale can be administered either over the phone or in-person as a brief questionnaire. **Table 1** reviews the different Frailty Scales and Indices. The accumulation of deficit approach does lend itself to screening either during patient history taking or via electronic medical records. The frailty index (FI) first developed by Rockwood, includes assessing for 70 deficits in different organ systems.[14,17] When Rockwood compared his 2 methods, the Clinical Frailty Scale versus the FI in the Canadian Study of Health and Aging (CSHA) database, he found that the clinical frailty scale was easier to operationalize but the FI allowed adverse risk outcomes to be defined more precisely. Since the CSHA FI, other accumulation of deficit instruments have been developed, including the American College of Surgeons National Surgical Improvement Program (ACS-NSQIP) 11-point modified frailty index (mFI), ACS-NSQIP 5-point mFI, European Prospective Investigation into Cancer, and Nutrition-Potsdam Frailty Index.[18–21] The current ACS-NSQIP 5-point mFI has a maximum of 5 points. Patients receive one point for each of the following: (1) functional health status partially or totally dependent, (2) diabetes (noninsulin or insulin dependent), (3) history of chronic obstructive pulmonary disease (COPD) or current pneumonia, (4) congestive heart failure within 30 days, and (5) hypertension requiring medication.[19] This scale has been repeatedly found to be predictive of postoperative complications from the ACS-NSQIP database in a wide variety of surgeries. This 5 element mFI is especially amenable to be asked during a routine preoperative review of systems either through a questionnaire, over the phone, or in-person. Unfortunately, these frailty assessments do not include an assessment of cognition. Screening for cognitive impairment must be performed in addition to frailty screening to determine cognitive frailty.

Intervening on frailty before surgery is an emerging area of research. Patients identified as frail could be referred for a comprehensive geriatric assessment (CGA). A geriatric specialist performing a CGA assesses the complex interaction of a multitude of medical problems, frailty, nutritional status, psychological and social statuses, and modifiable risk factors. CGA can identify high-risk medications, including deliriogenic

Table 1
Frailty instruments

Instrument	Elements Tested	Scoring	Requires In-Person
FRAIL Scale[13]	5 Elements Fatigue: Have you been fatigued all or most of the time in the past 4 weeks? Resistance: Do you have difficulty walking up 10 steps without an aide? Ambulation: Do you have difficulty walking a few hundred yards/meters without aids? Illnesses: Do you have more than 4 medical conditions? Loss of weight: Has the patient lost 5% or more weight in the past year?	1 point for each element 0: Robust 1–2: Prefrail 3–5: Frail	No
Clinical Frailty Scale[14]	Clinical Judgment ranging from very fit to severely frail: 1. Very fit = Robust, active, exercise regularly 2. Well = no active disease, exercise or are active occasionally 3. Managing well = controlled medical problems, not regularly active beyond routine walking 4. Vulnerable = Not dependent for daily help, symptoms limit activities, slow 5. Mildly Frail = More slowly, need help in high order ADL 6. Moderately Frail = Need help with ADL, help with stairs, help with bathing	Score 1 through 7 based on comprehensive assessment and clinical judgement An adjudication should occur by a multidisciplinary team	Yes or extensive clinical knowledge of the patient and their medical history

Fraility Phenotype[11]	5 Elements Weight loss: 10lbs or ≥5% within the past year Exhaustion: feeling tired all the time Low physical activity: inability to walk or needing assistance to walk Slowness: ≥19 s on a timed up and go test Weakness: weak grip strength	1 point for each element 0: Robust 1–2: Prefrail 3–5: Frail	Yes
Gait Speed[15]	Measured gate speed over 4 m	Gait speed <0.8 m/s is Frail and <0.2 m/s is extreme frailty	Yes
Gérontopôle Frailty Screening	6 Questions answered by provider: 1. Does your patient live alone? 2. Has your patient lost weight in the last 3 months? 3. Has your patient found it more difficult to get around in the past 3 months? 4. Does your patient complain of memory problems? 5. Does your patient have a slow gate speed (>4 s for 4 m)?	If provider answers yes to any question, they are then to ask themselves, "Do you think your patient is frail?" Then the patient is asked if they agree to a comprehensive frailty assessment	Yes
ACS-NSQIP 5 element mFI	5 elements to assess from interview or medical record 1. Functional health status is partially or totally dependent 2. Diabetes (noninsulin or insulin dependent) 3. History of COPD or current pneumonia 4. Congestive heart failure within 30 d 5. Hypertension requiring medication	Ordinal variable from 0 to1. Calculated as number of positive elements divided number of elements assessed. Cut offs: 0 = Robust 0.2–0.4 = Prefrail 0.6–1 = Frail	No

(continued on next page)

Table 1
(continued)

Instrument	Elements Tested	Scoring	Requires In-Person
ACS NSQIP 11 element mFI	11 elements assessed 1–5 of ACSONSQIP 5 element mFI 6. History of MI within the past 5 months before surgery 7. Previous percutaneous coronary intervention or cardiac surgery 8. Impaired sensorium 9. Transient ischemic attack 10. Stroke 11. Peripheral vascular disease with revascularization, amputation or rest pain	Analyzed as an ordinal variable with stepwise increases from 0 through 0.09, 0.18, 0.27, 0.36, 0.45, 0.54, 0.63, 0.72, 0.81, and 1.0	No
CSHA FI	70 elements over all domains and organ systems	Ordinal variable from 0 to1. Calculated as number of positive elements divided number of elements assessed	No, but requires extensive clinical knowledge of the patient and their medical history

medications, and allow for safe tapering. CGA can also identify if a patient may benefit from preoperative nutritional optimization or prehabilitation.[22] There is equipoise in the literature regarding whether a CGA can reduce a patient's risk of delirium. A recent meta-analysis investigated the effect of a CGA on POD and found that of 6 studies (n = 1611), 3 had a significant reduction in delirium, and 3 did not.[23] The pooled meta-analysis showed no significant difference in patients who had a CGA and those who did not (OR 0.76 [95% CI 0.30–1.96]). However, when only randomized controlled trials were included, there was a significant reduction in delirium in patients with a CGA intervention compared with the control group (OR 0.45 [95% CI 0.29–0.70]). The authors found the absolute risk reduction for the prevalence of delirium was 8.28% (95% CI 3.9–12.6), and the number needed to treat was 13 to prevent a case of delirium.[23] Adding frailty as an inclusion criterion to those who received a CGA could potentially further decrease the number to treat by focusing on a higher risk population. The CGA should also continue into the postoperative period with multidisciplinary teams executing evidence-based delirium prevention bundles such as Hospital Elder Life Program and the ICU Liberation bundles in frail older patients at heightened risk for delirium compared with their robust counterparts.[24,25]

TYPE OF ANESTHESIA AND POSTOPERATIVE DELIRIUM

Because there is no effective treatment of POD, identifying risk factors and preventive strategies is critically important. Many research studies have compared different anesthetic agents or various anesthetic modalities to identify a particular anesthetic method or drug that confers protection against POD. Identifying an anesthetic that is either protective or a risk factor could translate to changes in clinical practice that would stand to make a big difference in the outcomes of our older surgical patients. Here, we will briefly review recent literature comparing regional versus general anesthesia and the state of the evidence comparing the incidence of POD following total intravenous anesthesia (TIVA) versus inhalational anesthetics for maintenance of anesthesia.

Regional Versus General Anesthesia and Postoperative Delirium

Investigations comparing regional versus general anesthesia on the incidence of POD in older surgical patients date back to the 1980s. A common hypothesis was that regional anesthesia would decrease the incidence of delirium by avoiding general anesthetics that target the central nervous system to produce loss of consciousness, amnesia, and analgesia. Many anesthetic agents and other medications concomitantly administered during general anesthesia have been shown to have neurotoxic, neuroinflammatory, or anticholinergic effects. Alternatively, regional anesthesia can provide adequate surgical anesthesia without the need for loss of consciousness while also avoiding other potentially deliriogenic medications such as antiemetics or cholinergic agents. However, after decades of observational studies, randomized trials, meta-analyses, and systematic reviews, the evidence was never strong enough to support the choice of regional over general anesthesia for older surgical patients to prevent POD.

Many investigations and scientific reviews focused on patients having surgical hip fracture repair because this operation is commonly performed under either general or regional anesthesia and this is an older patient population in which POD is a common complication. Multiple systematic reviews and meta-analyses suggested no significant difference in the incidence of delirium between the 2 groups.[26] One common criticism of the studies comparing regional versus general anesthesia is the common use of sedation in the regional group. In these cases, it is not uncommon for patients to receive deep sedation with propofol and other anesthetic agents as an adjunct to the regional anesthetic. The criticism is that the varying levels of sedation could confound study results.

In 2010, a systematic review and meta-analysis included 21 trials investigating the incidence of either POD or postoperative cognitive dysfunction (POCD). There was no effect of anesthesia type on the odds ratio of developing either POD or POCD.[27] In 2016, a Cochrane Review comparing regional versus general anesthesia for hip fracture surgery in adults included an "acute confusional state" as an outcome. Based on 6 studies including 624 participants, there was no difference in the risk of acute confusional state: relative risk (RR) 0.85, 95% CI 0.51 to 1.40; $I^2 = 49\%$.[28]

Until recently, the available evidence had been limited to observational studies or very small clinical trials. In 2021, the results of 2 large, multicenter, randomized controlled trials comparing regional and general anesthesia for hip fracture surgery were published. The Regional versus General Anesthesia for Promoting Independence after Hip Fracture trial was a multicenter, pragmatic, randomized superiority trial that enrolled a total of 1600 patients with a mean age of 78 years.[29] The primary outcome was a composite of death and the inability to walk independently at 60 days postoperatively. POD was a secondary outcome. The investigators found that spinal anesthesia was not superior to general anesthesia with regard to survival, recovery of ambulation, and POD. The incidence of delirium was similar in the 2 groups occurring in 20.5% of the spinal anesthesia group and 19.7% in the general anesthesia group (RR 1.04; 95% CI 0.84–1.30). Of note, there was no limitation of the use of sedative agents in the regional anesthesia group.

The RAGA (Regional Anesthesia vs General Anesthesia) trial was a pragmatic, randomized, multicenter trial at university teaching hospitals in southeastern China that randomized 950 patients of mean age 76.5 years.[30] The primary outcome of RAGA was the incidence of delirium during the first 7 days postoperatively. Secondary outcomes included delirium severity, duration, and subtype. One unique aspect of the RAGA trial is that the patients randomized to regional anesthesia did not receive any sedation. Patients randomized to the regional group received a spinal, epidural, or combination of the two. Even in the absence of sedation, regional anesthesia did not significantly decrease the incidence of delirium compared with general anesthesia. POD occurred in 6.2% of the regional anesthesia group compared with 5.1% in the general anesthesia group (RR, 1.2 [95% CI, 0.7 to 2.0]; $P = .57$]). There were no differences between delirium severity scores or delirium subtype between groups.[30]

In 2022, a systematic review and meta-analysis aimed solely to determine whether general versus regional anesthesia was associated with POD incidence. The analysis included 21 relevant studies encompassing a total of more than 1.7 million patients. The pooled result of the meta-analysis found a significantly higher incidence of delirium after general anesthesia when compared to regional anesthesia (OR = 1.15, 95% CI: [1.02, 1.31], $I^2 = 83\%$, P for effect = .02). However, after removing 6 studies that were the main sources of high heterogeneity, a post hoc meta-analysis found no difference in POD between the 2 groups (OR = 0.95, 95% CI: [0.83, 1.08], $I^2 = 13\%$, P for effect = .44).[31]

A recent population-based cohort study compared dementia incidence in patients receiving different anesthetic types for hip fracture surgery. In a group of 268,014, the incidence was highest with general inhalational anesthesia. The incidence rate for inhalational versus regional anesthesia was 1.51 (1.15–1.66) and for TIVA versus regional anesthesia was 1.28 (1.09–1.51).[32]

Intravenous Versus Inhalational Anesthesia and Postoperative Delirium

General anesthesia is maintained with inhalational agents in up to 90% of surgeries[33]; however, maintenance by infusion of intravenous agents, primarily propofol, is a technique with potential advantages in the geriatric population. No consensus exists regarding the use of inhalational anesthesia versus TIVA to prevent POD in older adults. A recent Cochrane meta-analysis found a lack of conclusive evidence to differentiate TIVA versus inhalational anesthesia in the risk of POD. This is not surprising given the limited number of rigorous clinical trials, the small sample size in each study, frequently inadequate randomization, high attrition or selective reporting bias, imprecise or insensitive tools to measure delirium and cognition, and/or brevity of follow-up.[34]

Recently funded pragmatic, multicenter randomized controlled trials spanning the globe are set to answer the question of "Which is superior? IV or GAS?" VAPOR-C trial (Volatile Anaesthesia and Perioperative Outcomes Related to Cancer) is a study of intravenous versus volatile anesthetics on the duration of disease-free survival in patients with cancer.[35] VITAL (Volatile vs Total intravenous Anaesthesia for major noncardiac surgery: A pragmatic randomized triaL) will compare survival, safety, and cost-effectiveness of volatile anesthetic base anesthesia with TIVA in adults aged 50 years or older.[36] THRIVE (Trajectories of Recovery after Intravenous Propofol vs inhaled VolatilE anesthesia) focuses on the quality of recovery on postoperative day 1 and has a safety outcome of intraoperative awareness.[37] We eagerly await the results of these trials that are poised to be landmark studies in anesthesiology.

DELIRIUM AND LONG-TERM COGNITION

Delirium is described as an acute attentional deficit, which waxes and wanes. The natural course of POD is that it improves as the patient's health status improves. Although POD seems transient, it is associated with increased health-care costs, a longer length of stay, morbidity, and mortality. The literature has primarily focused on in-hospital delirium and less on long-term (months and years) cognitive trajectory. Studies of long-term cognition are more difficult to perform; they require out of hospital follow-up, extended study visits, and significant costs for personnel and training. More recently, large studies have described in detail the cognitive performance and trajectory of physical recovery that are vitally important to patients and the health-care system.

The International Study of Postoperative Cognitive Dysfunction was one of the largest early studies of delirium and POCD. In 2008, this study group published data demonstrating an early (7-day) relationship between POD and cognitive dysfunction but did not find a relationship 3 months after surgery. The authors commented that the study was underpowered due to the dropout of what may have been the most vulnerable population. In 2016, The Successful Aging after Elective Surgery (SAGES) group published a study examining cognitive trajectory in patients who did and did not develop POD. They used more in-depth cognitive measures and longer term follow-up and showed a clear decline in postoperative cognitive ability after adjusting for cognitive baseline in a larger (556 person) group followed up for 18 months.[38] The objective decline on cognitive testing was in agreement with the performance as described by patients' families using the Informant Questionnaire on Cognitive Decline in the Elderly measure.[39] In fact, the rate of cognitive decline after an episode of POD was similar to patients who have a diagnosis of mild cognitive impairment[40,41]; significantly faster than normal aging although slower than frank dementia. The same group demonstrated that patients with mild cognitive impairment who have an episode of delirium had worsened cognitive decline after surgery compared with patients with mild cognitive impairment who do not have an episode of delirium.[42]

In 2018, a study of ICU patients examined the association between the cause of a delirium episode (ie, sedative-associated, hypoxic, septic) and long-term cognitive outcomes. They found that delirium from any cause was associated with worse long-term cognition 12 months after hospital discharge, even after adjustment for common confounders such as age, comorbidity, preoperative cognition, and education.[43] The authors noted that these findings are particularly significant because even delirium associated with sedative administration is associated with worse long-term cognition.

The relationship between delirium and long-term cognitive disorders does not belie a relationship between general anesthesia and surgery (per se) and long-term cognitive decline. Whitlock and colleagues[44] published a study that compared cognitive trajectory for patients who had coronary artery bypass graft surgery (CABG) versus percutaneous coronary intervention (PCI) as measured by a summary measure of cognitive tests in the Health and Retirement study, called the memory score. They found that the cognitive trajectory during 10 years was the same for both groups of patients. This suggests that even major surgery and general anesthesia do not "cause" cognitive decline. It is important to note that they did identify a group of patients who developed major neurocognitive disorders after either CABG or PCI. The reason for long-term cognitive function in this study was not identified, and the role of delirium was not investigated because the study used a large dataset that did not collect delirium screening for all patients.

A Mechanistic Review of Delirium and Dementia

A recent review article by Drs Fong and Inouye described the interrelationship between delirium and dementia.[45] Patients with dementia more often develop delirium, and as we mentioned, delirium is associated with accelerated cognitive decline. The article summarized the evidence for the mechanism behind both conditions with respect to shared biomarkers, systemic inflammation, neuroinflammation, Alzheimer disease biomarkers, Apolipoprotein E, and functional connectivity. Systemic and neuroinflammation have both been associated with POD. Which inflammatory markers are associated and at what time point (before surgery) versus after surgery has also been described. Some cytokines have been identified as risk factors, and others as markers of disease severity. The Successful Aging After Elective Surgery Study (SAGES) performed a case-control study of patients aged older than 70 years undergoing major noncardiac surgery who did and did not develop delirium.[46] They found that preoperative c-reactive protein (CRP) is a "risk marker" for POD. A preoperative CRP level of 3 mg/L or greater was associated with a 1.5 times greater risk of developing delirium than patients with lower levels of CRP. Other markers of the nuclear factor kappa B pathway are markers for delirium, although they tend to be elevated at the time of delirium. This led the Vasunilashorn group to suggest they are "disease markers." For example, this is the case for cytokines such as interleukin (IL) 6, IL 2, vascular endothelial growth factor, and tumor necrosis factor-alpha (TNFα) at postoperative day 2.[47] A meta-analysis of delirium and inflammation published in 2021 identified 17 studies with a low risk of bias and found that preoperative IL6 and CRP were associated with POD.[48] The meta-analysis did not find evidence for an association of POD with IL8, IL10, TNFα, or insulin-like growth factor (IGF)-1. There was a lack of preoperative association between cortisol and POD; however, the authors commented that the issue of diurnal variation with cortisol might have confounded the findings.

Regarding the association between dementia and delirium, studies suggest that patients with dementia are more susceptible to the deliriogenic effects of inflammation. There is also evidence to suggest that pathways such as neuroinflammation influence the progression of Alzheimer's dementia.[49] Presence of apolipoprotein E4 (Apo E4) allele is a risk factor for dementia but has a less clear association with delirium. Patients with the Apo E4 allele may have a heterogeneous response to inflammation with respect to the development of delirium than patients without the allele.[50–52] Preoperative elevated serum neurofilament light (NfL), a marker for axonal damage, has been associated with POD.[53] The same study demonstrated that elevated NfL at 1 month after surgery is also associated with cognitive decline. This may be evidence for axonal damage as part of the mechanism that links POD and cognitive decline. Dementia and delirium are also both associated with blood–brain barrier (BBB) disruption. One study looked at BBB disruption in a cohort of older hip fracture patients. They found BBB disruption in patients with and without dementia; however, all patients with BBB disruption experienced delirium or subsyndromal delirium.[54]

DELIRIUM AND FUNCTIONAL RECOVERY

POD has been found to be associated with worse functional recovery in older surgical patients. In 2000, a study of 126 hip fracture patients who underwent emergent surgery described that delirium was associated with poor functional recovery 1 month later even after adjustment for preoperative cognition and functional status. These outcomes included activities of daily living (ADL) decline, a decline in ambulation, and death or new nursing home placement.[55] Subsequently, in 2017, a large cohort of 556 patients undergoing elective surgery showed that those who experienced delirium had lesser functional recovery up to 18 months after surgery.[56] For this study, function was measured as a composite of the ADLS, Instrumental Activity of Daily Living, and the physical component of the Short Form-12 (SF-12). More studies are needed to measure functional and patient-centered outcomes in older surgical patients months and years after surgery.

SUMMARY

POD is not a benign or inert process and may be a modifiable risk factor for dementia. The immediate complications from delirium, such as falls, increased health-care costs, and patient-centered outcomes are familiar. The current data supports that delirium is associated with long-term cognitive decline and dementia. Given the magnitude of the older surgical population and the high incidence, POD is a major public health concern. Several states, such as Massachusetts and New Hampshire, mandated that hospitals implement plans for delirium recognition and prevention. Given the magnitude and severity of delirium and its consequences, these measures are a great starting place but are not adequate. Additional mandates to encourage best practices for delirium prevention will likely evolve in the future as the prevention of delirium gains recognition as a public health priority.

CLINICS CARE POINTS

- Frailty differs from healthy aging. Healthy aging is accompanied by physiologic changes but these changes do not lead to the severe depletion of reserve and vulnerability even to small stressors.

- Frailty can be screened and diagnosed by various validated instruments.
- Example instruments include FRAIL (Fatigue, Resistance, Ambulation, Illness, Loss of weight) scale, the Clinical Frailty Scale, the Frailty Phenotype, Gait Speed, and the Gérontopôle Frailty Screening Tool.
- A recent meta-analysis found that when only randomized clinical trials were included, there was a significant reduction in delirium in patients with a Comprehensive Geriatric Assessment (CGA) intervention compared with the control group (OR 0.45 [95% CI 0.29–0.70]).
- Recent multicenter, randomized controlled trials comparing regional and general anesthesia for hip fracture surgery found no differences in the incidence of delirium between groups.

DISCLOSURE

Dr Deiner is a director for the ABA; opinions expressed in this paper do not represent the views of the ABA. She has been an expert witness. She has had no industry relationships for >5 years. Drs Mahanna-Gabrielli and Schenning have no conflicts of interest.

FUNDING

Katie J. Schenning is funded by the National Institute on Aging K76-AG074938.

REFERENCES

1. Brivio P, Paladini MS, Racagni G, et al. From healthy aging to frailty: in search of the underlying mechanisms. Curr Med Chem 2019;26(20):3685–701.
2. Sugimoto T, Arai H, Sakurai T. An update on cognitive frailty: Its definition, impact, associated factors and underlying mechanisms, and interventions. Geriatr Gerontol Int 2022;22(2):99–109.
3. Kelaiditi E, Cesari M, Canevelli M, et al. Cognitive frailty: rational and definition from an (I.A.N.A./I.A.G.G.) international consensus group. J Nutr Health Aging 2013;17(9):726–34.
4. Cesari M, Andrieu S, Rolland Y, et al. The cognitive impairment of frail older persons. J Nutr Health Aging 2013;17(9):735–7.
5. Delrieu J, Andrieu S, Pahor M, et al. Neuropsychological profile of "cognitive frailty" subjects in MAPT study. J Prev Alzheimers Dis 2016;3(3):151–9.
6. Hoogendijk EO, Afilalo J, Ensrud KE, et al. Frailty: implications for clinical practice and public health. Lancet 2019;394(10206):1365–75.
7. Panza F, Lozupone M, Solfrizzi V, et al. Different cognitive frailty models and health- and cognitive-related outcomes in older age: from epidemiology to prevention. J Alzheimers Dis 2018;62(3):993–1012.
8. Gracie TJ, Caufield-Noll C, Wang NY, et al. The association of preoperative frailty and postoperative delirium: a meta-analysis. Anesth Analg 2021;133(2):314–23.
9. Fu D, Tan X, Zhang M, et al. Association between frailty and postoperative delirium: a meta-analysis of cohort study. Aging Clin Exp Res 2022;34(1):25–37.
10. Zhang XM, Jiao J, Xie XH, et al. The association between frailty and delirium among hospitalized patients: an updated meta-analysis. J Am Med Dir Assoc 2021;22(3):527–34.
11. Fried LP, Tangen CM, Walston J, et al. Frailty in older adults: evidence for a phenotype. J Gerontol A Biol Sci Med Sci 2001;56(3):M146–56.

12. Mitnitski AB, Mogilner AJ, Rockwood K. Accumulation of deficits as a proxy measure of aging. Sci World J 2001;1:323–36.

13. Abellan van Kan G, Rolland Y, Bergman H, et al. The I.A.N.A Task Force on frailty assessment of older people in clinical practice. J Nutr Health Aging 2008;12(1): 29–37.

14. Rockwood K, Song X, MacKnight C, et al. A global clinical measure of fitness and frailty in elderly people. CMAJ (Can Med Assoc J) 2005;173(5):489–95.

15. Abellan van Kan G, Rolland Y, Andrieu S, et al. Gait speed at usual pace as a predictor of adverse outcomes in community-dwelling older people an International Academy on Nutrition and Aging (IANA) Task Force. J Nutr Health Aging 2009;13(10):881–9.

16. Subra J, Gillette-Guyonnet S, Cesari M, et al. The integration of frailty into clinical practice: preliminary results from the Gérontopôle. J Nutr Health Aging 2012; 16(8):714–20.

17. Rockwood K, Andrew M, Mitnitski A. A comparison of two approaches to measuring frailty in elderly people. J Gerontol A Biol Sci Med Sci 2007;62(7): 738–43.

18. Velanovich V, Antoine H, Swartz A, et al. Accumulating deficits model of frailty and postoperative mortality and morbidity: its application to a national database. J Surg Res 2013;183(1):104–10.

19. Subramaniam S, Aalberg JJ, Soriano RP, et al. New 5-Factor modified frailty index using american college of surgeons NSQIP data. J Am Coll Surg 2018;226(2): 173–81.e178.

20. Subramaniam S, Aalberg JJ, Soriano RP, et al. The 5-factor modified frailty index in the geriatric surgical population. Am Surg 2021;87(9):1420–5.

21. Lachmann R, Stelmach-Mardas M, Bergmann MM, et al. The accumulation of deficits approach to describe frailty. PLoS One 2019;14(10):e0223449.

22. Zietlow KE, Wong S, Heflin MT, et al. Geriatric preoperative optimization: a review. Am J Med 2022;135(1):39–48.

23. Saripella A, Wasef S, Nagappa M, et al. Effects of comprehensive geriatric care models on postoperative outcomes in geriatric surgical patients: a systematic review and meta-analysis. BMC Anesthesiol 2021;21(1):127.

24. Pun BT, Balas MC, Barnes-Daly MA, et al. Caring for critically Ill patients with the ABCDEF bundle: results of the ICU liberation collaborative in over 15,000 adults. Crit Care Med 2019;47(1):3–14.

25. Hshieh TT, Yang T, Gartaganis SL, et al. Hospital elder life program: systematic review and meta-analysis of effectiveness. Am J Geriatr Psychiatry 2018; 26(10):1015–33.

26. O'Donnell CM, McLoughlin L, Patterson CC, et al. Perioperative outcomes in the context of mode of anaesthesia for patients undergoing hip fracture surgery: systematic review and meta-analysis. Br J Anaesth 2018;120(1):37–50.

27. Mason SE, Noel-Storr A, Ritchie CW. The impact of general and regional anesthesia on the incidence of post-operative cognitive dysfunction and post-operative delirium: a systematic review with meta-analysis. J Alzheim Dis : JAD. 2010; 22(Suppl 3):67–79.

28. Guay J, Parker MJ, Gajendragadkar PR, et al. Anaesthesia for hip fracture surgery in adults. Cochrane Database Syst Rev 2016;2(2):CD000521.

29. Neuman MD, Feng R, Carson JL, et al. Spinal anesthesia or general anesthesia for hip surgery in older adults. N Engl J Med 2021;385(22):2025–35.

30. Li T, Li J, Yuan L, et al. Effect of regional vs general anesthesia on incidence of postoperative delirium in older patients undergoing hip fracture surgery: the RAGA randomized trial. JAMA 2022;327(1):50–8.

31. Zhu X, Yang M, Mu J, et al. The effect of general anesthesia vs. regional anesthesia on postoperative delirium-a systematic review and meta-analysis. Front Med 2022;9:844371.

32. Sun M, Chen WM, Wu SY, et al. Dementia risk amongst older adults with hip fracture receiving general anaesthesia or regional anaesthesia: a propensity-score-matched population-based cohort study. Br J Anaesth 2023 Mar;130(3):305–13.

33. Pandit JJ, Andrade J, Bogod DG, et al. 5th National Audit Project (NAP5) on accidental awareness during general anaesthesia: summary of main findings and risk factors. Br J Anaesth 2014;113(4):549–59.

34. Miller D, Lewis SR, Pritchard MW, et al. Intravenous versus inhalational maintenance of anaesthesia for postoperative cognitive outcomes in elderly people undergoing non-cardiac surgery, *Cochrane Database Syst Rev* . 2018 Aug 21;8(8):CD012317.

35. Dubowitz JA, Cata JP, De Silva AP, et al. Volatile anaesthesia and peri-operative outcomes related to cancer: a feasibility and pilot study for a large randomised control trial. Anaesthesia 2021;76(9):1198–206.

36. ISRCTN62903453, VITAL: a trial looking at which general anaesthesia technique is better for patient recovery following major non-cardiac surgery. BMC. 2021. Available at: https://www.isrctn.com/ISRCTNISRCTN62903453. Accessed 2021 Oct 10.

37. THRIVE: Trajectories of Recovery after Intravenous Propofol vs inhaled VolatilE anesthesia. Patient-Centered Outcomes Research Institute. 2021. Available at: https://www.pcori.org/research-results/2021/thrive-trajectories-recovery-after-intravenous-propofol-vs-inhaled-volatile. Accessed August 9, 2021.

38. Inouye SK, Marcantonio ER, Kosar CM, et al. The short-term and long-term relationship between delirium and cognitive trajectory in older surgical patients. Alzheimers Dement 2016;12(7):766–75.

39. Jorm AF, Scott R, Cullen JS, et al. Performance of the Informant Questionnaire on Cognitive Decline in the Elderly (IQCODE) as a screening test for dementia. Psychol Med 1991;21(3):785–90.

40. Johnson JK, Gross AL, Pa J, et al. Longitudinal change in neuropsychological performance using latent growth models: a study of mild cognitive impairment. Brain Imaging Behav 2012;6(4):540–50.

41. Hayden KM, Reed BR, Manly JJ, et al. Cognitive decline in the elderly: an analysis of population heterogeneity. Age Ageing 2011;40(6):684–9.

42. Racine AM, Fong TG, Gou Y, et al. Clinical outcomes in older surgical patients with mild cognitive impairment. Alzheimers Dement 2018;14(5):590–600.

43. Girard TD, Thompson JL, Pandharipande PP, et al. Clinical phenotypes of delirium during critical illness and severity of subsequent long-term cognitive impairment: a prospective cohort study. Lancet Respir Med 2018;6(3):213–22.

44. Whitlock EL, Diaz-Ramirez LG, Smith AK, et al. Association of coronary artery bypass grafting vs percutaneous coronary intervention with memory decline in older adults undergoing coronary revascularization. JAMA 2021;325(19):1955–64.

45. Fong TG, Inouye SK. The inter-relationship between delirium and dementia: the importance of delirium prevention. Nat Rev Neurol 2022;18(10):579–96.

46. Vasunilashorn SM, Ngo L, Inouye SK, et al. Cytokines and postoperative delirium in older patients undergoing major elective surgery. J Gerontol A Biol Sci Med Sci 2015;70(10):1289–95.
47. Vasunilashorn SM, Ngo LH, Chan NY, et al. Development of a dynamic multi-protein signature of postoperative delirium. J Gerontol A Biol Sci Med Sci 2019; 74(2):261–8.
48. De Jongh RF, Vissers KC, Meert TF, et al. The role of interleukin-6 in nociception and pain. Anesth Analg 2003;96(4):1096–103.
49. Leng F, Edison P. Neuroinflammation and microglial activation in Alzheimer disease: where do we go from here? Nat Rev Neurol 2021;17(3):157–72.
50. Ely EW, Girard TD, Shintani AK, et al. Apolipoprotein E4 polymorphism as a genetic predisposition to delirium in critically ill patients. Crit Care Med 2007; 35(1):112–7.
51. Leung JM, Sands LP, Wang Y, et al. Apolipoprotein E e4 allele increases the risk of early postoperative delirium in older patients undergoing noncardiac surgery. Anesthesiology 2007;107(3):406–11.
52. van Munster BC, Korevaar JC, Zwinderman AH, et al. The association between delirium and the apolipoprotein E epsilon 4 allele: new study results and a meta-analysis. Am J Geriatr Psychiatry 2009;17(10):856–62.
53. Fong TG, Vasunilashorn SM, Ngo L, et al. Association of plasma neurofilament light with postoperative delirium. Ann Neurol 2020;88(5):984–94.
54. Hov KR, Berg JP, Frihagen F, et al. Blood-cerebrospinal fluid barrier integrity in delirium determined by Q-albumin. Dement Geriatr Cogn Disord 2016;41(3–4): 192–8.
55. Marcantonio ER, Flacker JM, Michaels M, et al. Delirium is independently associated with poor functional recovery after hip fracture. J Am Geriatr Soc 2000;48(6): 618–24.
56. Hshieh TT, Saczynski J, Gou RY, et al. Trajectory of functional recovery after postoperative delirium in elective surgery. Ann Surg 2017;265(4):647–53.

Mechanical Circulatory Support Devices in the Elderly

Bhoumesh Patel, MD[a],*, Robert P. Davis, MD[b],
Siavosh Saatee, MD[c]

KEYWORDS

- Mechanical circulatory support • Cardiogenic shock • Elderly • Geriatrics • Frailty

KEY POINTS

- Because mechanical circulatory support (MCS) continues to advance with improving outcomes, elderly patients previously not considered for MCS are now being supported.
- All MCS devices, to varying degrees, restore systemic circulation, improve oxygen delivery, reduce ventricular distension, thereby reducing wall stress, stroke work, and myocardial oxygen consumption.
- Extracorporeal membrane oxygenation should be considered earlier in the clinical course of the disease and initiated without a delay before prolonged hypoperfusion leads to a significant degree of metabolic derangement.
- Palliative care physician should be consulted throughout the course MCS therapy, from decision-making period, preimplantation, through the duration of MCS therapy.
- Age itself should not preclude patients from being candidates for MCS.

INTRODUCTION

Mechanical circulatory support (MCS) era began in 1953 with the development of cardiopulmonary bypass to facilitate open-heart surgery.[1] Past few decades have seen substantial progress in MCS, and it has expanded the treatment options for patients. Currently available MCS devices can be implanted percutaneously or surgically. They can also be configured to support the left, right, or both ventricles, offering varying levels of circulatory support.[2] Because the field continues to advance and resuscitation protocols are being refined, patients previously not considered for MCS are now being

[a] Division of Cardiac Anesthesiology, Department of Anesthesiology, Yale School of Medicine, 333 Cedar Street, P.O. Box 208051, New Haven, CT 06520-8051, USA; [b] Division of Cardiac Surgery, Department of Surgery, Yale School of Medicine, 333 Cedar Street, P.O. Box 208051, New Haven, CT 06520-8051, USA; [c] Department of Anesthesiology, Feinberg School of Medicine, 251 East Huron St., F5-704, Chicago, IL 60611, USA
* Correspondence author.
E-mail address: bhoumesh.patel@yale.edu

Anesthesiology Clin 41 (2023) 583–594
https://doi.org/10.1016/j.anclin.2023.02.008
1932-2275/23/© 2023 Elsevier Inc. All rights reserved.
anesthesiology.theclinics.com

supported. An elderly patient is defined as having a chronological age of 65 years or older. However, there is no clear medical or biological evidence to support this definition. Many of the elderly patients, especially those aged younger than 75 years, are still robust and active. During the last century, life expectancy has increased, and population ageing is a global phenomenon. In the United States, for example, this increased from 47.3 years at birth in 1900 to 78.7 years in 2010.[3] According to the latest population estimates and projections from UN Department of Economic and Social Affairs's Population Division, 1 in 6 people in the world will be aged older than 65 years by 2050, up from 1 in 11 in 2019.[4] In many regions, the population aged 65 years will double by 2050, whereas global life expectancy beyond 65 years will increase by 19 years.[4] Currently, there are no published guidelines for the use of MCS in the elderly. The purpose of our review is to provide anesthesiologists caring for elderly patients with an overview of commonly use MCS and discuss fundamental principles of these devices, physiological effect, elderly specific factors when considering MCS.

Mechanical Circulatory Support Devices and Hemodynamic Effects

MCS devices can broadly be classified based on duration of support into temporary or durable devices. Patients with durable devices can be discharged from the hospital. Temporary MCS devices can be placed percutaneously or surgically but patient on these cannot leave the hospital. In addition, these devices can be used in various configurations, alone or in combination with each other to support either right, left, or both ventricles.

Mechanical circulatory support devices for right ventricular failure

Right ventricular failure remains a major cause of morbidity and mortality.[5] MCS devices for the RV are an important tool in the management of cardiogenic shock due to RV failure with the ability to rapidly stabilize patients and restore perfusion. The most used devices are the intra-aortic balloon pump (IABP), the Impella RP (AbioMed, Danvers, MA), the TandemHeart (LivaNova, London, England, UK), and venoarterial extracorporeal membrane oxygenation (VA-ECMO; **Fig. 1**).

Mechanical circulatory support devices for left ventricular failure

Left ventricular mechanical support devices can be broadly classified based on the hemodynamic circuit as (A) left ventricle (LV) to aorta assist devices, namely, the IABP and the Impella; (B) left atrium (LA) to systemic artery, namely, the Tandem Heart; and (C) the right atrium (RA) to systemic artery, namely, venoarterial extracorporeal membrane oxygenation (VA-ECMO; **Fig. 2**).

Mechanical Circulatory Support Devices Physiology and Hemodynamic Effects

All MCS devices, to varying degrees, restore systemic circulation, improve oxygen delivery, reduce ventricular distension, thereby reducing wall stress, stroke work, and myocardial oxygen consumption.[2,6,7] However, the specific features such as circuit configurations, flow rates, and characteristics of the pump (eg, axial, or centrifugal flow) result in different overall cardiac and systemic hemodynamic effects.[6–8] In addition, baseline volume status, myocardial function, and systemic vascular resistance determines the response of a given patient to a specific MCS device. Therefore, it is of utmost importance to differentiate between the primary hemodynamic effects of a device and the net hemodynamic changes observed.

Intra-aortic balloon pump

IABP augments pulsatile blood flow by inflating during diastole, increasing mean aortic pressure, thereby improving coronary perfusion. Balloon deflation during systole

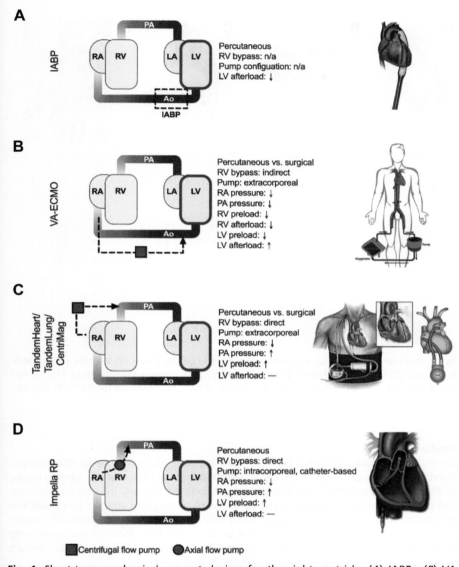

Fig. 1. Short-term mechanical support devices for the right ventricle. (*A*) IABPs; (*B*) VA-ECMO; (*C*) TandemHeart, TandemLung, and CentriMag devices; and (*D*) Impella RP. (Created with BioRender.com.)

reduces LV afterload, left ventricular end-diastolic pressure (LVEDP), right ventricular afterload, and myocardial oxygen demand.[7,9] Overall, it increases LV stroke volume, systemic mean arterial pressure, reduces left ventricular diastolic volume and pressure, and increases coronary perfusion pressure.[10] However, IABP does not directly improve flow, with typically causing only a modest increase in cardiac output of $\cong$ 0.5 L/min.[9,10] Hence, IABP largely is regarded as a means of augmenting coronary and systemic perfusion pressure and reducing LV dilation and pulmonary congestion, rather than an effective form of MCS (see **Fig. 1**).

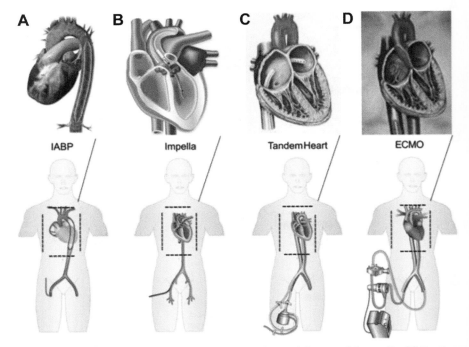

Fig. 2. Short-term mechanical support devices for the LV. (*A*) IABPs, (*B*) Impella, (*C*) Tandem-Heart, and (*D*) VA-ECMO. (*From* [Brown JL, Estep JD. Temporary Percutaneous Mechanical Circulatory Support in Advanced Heart Failure. Heart Fail Clin. 2016 Jul;12(3):385–98]; with permission.)

Impella

The Impella devices (Abiomed, Danvers, MA) are continuous microaxial flow pumps. Blood is pumped directly from the LV, independent of the phase of the cardiac cycle, resulting in the loss of the normal isovolumic periods. As a result, the pressure volume loop changes from its normal trapezoidal shape to a triangular shape.[2] It unloads the LV directly, leading to a decrease in the LVEDP and decreasing myocardial oxygen consumption.[2] By diverting blood into the aorta, it increases forward flow improving the systemic mean arterial blood pressure (**Fig. 3**). These pumps provide cardiac output augmentation ranging from 2.5 L/min up to 6 L/min.

Tandem heart system

The TandemHeart is a percutaneous device (Cardiac Assist, Inc; Pittsburgh, PA) is an extracorporeal LA to femoral artery bypass continuous flow centrifugal pump that can provide support of up to 4 L/min. Overall hemodynamic affect include increased cardiac output and unloading of the LV, resulting in a decrease in pulmonary artery occlusion pressure, pulmonary artery pressure, and reduced myocardial workload, and oxygen demand.[2,11] It requires adequate RV function to maintain left atrial volume. However, in the setting of worsening RV failure, it can be converted to an ECMO circuit by repositioning the inflow cannula back across the interatrial septum into the RA and adding a membrane oxygenator to the circuit to provide complete cardiopulmonary support.

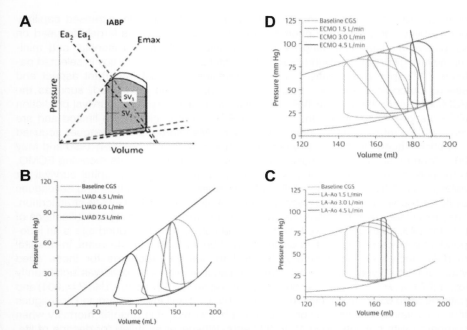

Fig. 3. Hemodynamics effect on pressure-volume loops. (*A*) IABP reduces peak LV systolic and diastolic pressures and increases LV stroke volume. (*B*) Pressure–volume loop with LV to aorta assist device such as the Impella, the LVEDP decreases and there is an increased uncoupling of the aortic and peak left ventricular pressure generation. (*C*) Pressure–volume loops with left atrial-to-aortic (LA-Ao) pumping such as Tandem Heart, showing reducing end-diastolic pressures, increasing end-systolic volume, and decreasing LV stroke volume. (*D*) Pressure–volume loop with VA-ECMO. Increasing flow is associated with an increase in the LVEDP, a decrease in LV stroke volume, and an increase in the effective arterial elastance. (*Adapted from* [Burkhoff D, Sayer G, Doshi D et al. Hemodynamic of Mechanical Circulatory Support. JACC, 2015 Dec;66(23):2663-2674; with permission and Rihal CS, Naidu SS, Givertz MM et al 2015 SCAI/ACC/HFSA/STS Clinical Expert Consensus Statement on the Use of Percutaneous Mechanical Circulatory Support Devices in Cardiovascular Care. JACC 2015 May 19;65(19):e7-e26)]; with permission.)

Extracorporeal membrane oxygenation

There are 2 types of extracorporeal support: the venovenous ECMO (VV-ECMO) that is used solely for pulmonary support and the VA-ECMO that provides total cardiopulmonary and biventricular support. The overall hemodynamic effect of VA-ECMO is increased global systemic perfusion and mean arterial pressure.[2] However, it causes increased LV afterload with subsequent increase in LVEDP and pulmonary capillary wedge pressure and decreased LV stroke volume.[2] This may lead to deleterious consequences and may exacerbate LV ischemia unless the LV is unloaded. LV can be decompressed with various strategies that include percutaneous options such as IABP, Impella, or atrial septostomy; surgical options such as direct LV apical or left atrial cannulation; or medical management that includes increasing inotropic support and vasodilation.[12]

Venovenous extracorporeal membrane oxygenation outcomes in the elderly. Acute respiratory distress syndrome (ARDS) is a life-threatening form of respiratory failure, characterized by acute inflammatory lung injury that results in increased capillary permeability and pulmonary edema.[13] Management of ARDS is largely focused on supportive management, lung-protective ventilation, prone positioning, and minimizing iatrogenic forms of lung injury with ECMO as a salvage therapy in selected patients.[14–16] Appropriate patient selection remains the most important aspect and several outcome prediction scoring systems have been developed, such as the ECMOnet score, the PRESERVE score, and the respiratory ecmo survival prediction (RESP) score.[17–19] Data on the use of VV-ECMO in the elderly are limited and are mostly from retrospective studies. A study by Mendiratta and colleagues focused on patients aged older than 65 years supported with ECMO between 1990 and May 2013 found a significant increase in the number of elderly patients receiving ECMO, with more than two-thirds of cases performed after 2010. In-hospital survival for elderly was 41%, compared with 55% for all other adults.[20] Deatrick and colleagues evaluated survival to hospital discharge for patients on VV-ECMO by age stratification. They examined the relationship between age and mortality with age stratifications of less than 45, 45 to 54, 55 to 64, and more than 65 years. They found age is an independent predictor of survival to discharge and beginning at age 45 years, in-hospital mortality increases incrementally. Survival to hospital discharge for those aged younger than 45 years was 84.6%, for those aged 45 years or older was significantly lower (67.0%; $P = .009$), as was survival for those aged 55 years (57.1%; $P = .001$) and patients aged 65 years or older (16.7%; $P = .003$).[21] Similarly, Barbaro and colleagues found increasing age was associated with a higher risk of in-hospital mortality when compared with patients aged 16 to 39 years. Whenever stratified for decade of life, this was progressive with a mortality hazard ratio of 1.76 (1.23–2.52) for those aged 50 to 59 years and as high as 3.07 (1.58–5.95) in patients aged older than 70 years.[22] Pranikoff and colleagues[23] found that survival was inversely correlated with the number of days of mechanical ventilation before ECMO. In that study, the predicted mortality rate was 50% after 5 days of mechanical ventilation.[23] Above data suggest that the older age alone should not be a contraindication and indicate that the initiation of ECMO support in elderly patients with respiratory failure should be considered and undertaken early in the clinical course without a delay before prolonged hypoxemia leads to a significant degree of metabolic derangement.

ST-elevation Myocardial Infarction and Mechanical Support

Percutaneous coronary intervention (PCI) remains to be the standard management of ST-elevation myocardial infarction (STEMI); however, there is lack of proper perfusion in about a third of patients after catheterization.[24] Moreover, there is evidence to suggest association with pre-PCI LV mechanical unloading with myocardial protection and augmented myocardial recovery.[25] LV unloading minimizes the reperfusion injury by decreasing the myocardial oxygen requirement, thus limiting ischemic/infarct size.[24,25] (Fig. 4) Increasing body of data suggest that pre-PCI LV mechanical unloading is associated with an improved survival.[26] Patients aged 75 years and older with STEMI are at higher risk to present in cardiogenic shock.[24] Other causes such as postcardiotomy cardiogenic shock, myocarditis, stress-induced cardiomyopathy, pulmonary embolization, and even a mixed picture of sepsis, bleeding, can manifest as cardiogenic shock and should be carefully distinguished. When shock persists, despite preload and afterload optimization, the need for more cardiac output is needed to avoid or recover from multiorgan failure. Temporary MCS should be initiated as soon as possible to stabilize the patient and avoid further deterioration from the initial insult. Moreover, it will create a window of opportunity for further thorough clinical assessment.

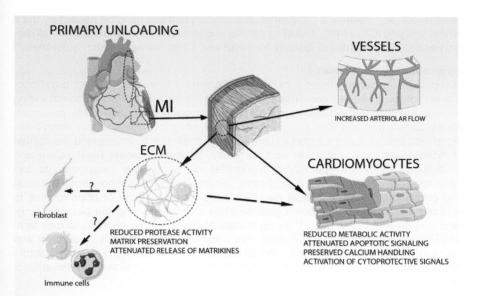

Fig. 4. Cellular mechanisms remediating the proposed protective effects of primary unloading in the infarcted heart. (*Source*: Hanna A, Frangogiannis NG. The cell biological basis for primary unloading in acute myocardial infarction. Int J Cardiol. 2019 Oct 15;293:45–47.)

Elderly Specific Considerations

Frailty

Frailty does not have a universally acceptable definition but has been generally defined as a condition that results from increased vulnerability to stressors. It has been reported to have affected up to 60% of patients with advanced heart failure and had been associated with increased mortality, prolonged length of stay, and prolonged time on the ventilator and time to hospital discharge in heart failure patients.[27,28]

Frailty evaluation involves the measurement of various deficits ranging from physical to cognitive and psychosocial aspects of patients. Some basic screening measures such as slow chair rise, slow gait and poor ambulation that highlights the need for assistance to complete basic daily tasks have been shown to independently increase the risks of perioperative mortality by 2 to 4 times, compared with nonfrail patients in cardiac procedures.[28]

Sarcopenia is defined as the age-related decline in skeletal muscle mass and strength and is the cornerstone of the frailty syndrome.[29] It is an objective variable (usually less than 2 standard deviation muscle mass of a healthy normal in men and women) is aimed to replace some subjective general measures such as weight loss and body mass index. Various imaging modalities have been proposed to measure sarcopenia.[30,31] Modalities such as dual x-ray absorptiometry scans, computed tomography (CT) scans, MRI, or bioimpedance testing are usually needed but CT imaging has been the one used and validated widely in cardiac surgeries, specially left ventricular assist device (LVAD) operations.[31,32]

Neurologic

Considering the higher risk of cognitive dysfunction, postoperative delirium, and the presence of other comorbidities such as dementia, unrecognized stroke, and cerebrovascular disease; a comprehensive examination seems to be necessary but a proper imaging (CT or MRI), including carotid and vertebral Doppler studies are all recommended by International Society for Heart and Lung Transplantation guidelines.[33]

Psychosocial considerations

Frail patients, especially those with advanced age have more neurological, psychosocial, and musculoskeletal comorbidities. That can impair their ability for understanding and communicating their desired goal of care and reasonable quality of life, postoperatively. Diminished cognitive and sensory ability in advanced age specially when combined with limited social support will create huge challenge to understand the burden of disease and care, medically and surgically. Patients in acute heart failure and cardiogenic shock are specially at higher risk of neurological derangements and have less time available for a long-term, proper decision-making communication and education. Temporary MCS provides a significant window of opportunities to evaluate and improve the neurological function while discussing the potential long-term durable MCS candidacy.[34] Being in state of shock, most patients and their families choose an aggressive approach that maximize their chances of survival and therefore would agree with any offered procedure at the time. However, factors such as depression and acceptance of their illness can result in significant dissatisfaction, usually 6 months after initiating LVAD education.[35]

Pulmonary

Although pulmonary function test (PFT) is not mandatory preoperatively for patients undergoing MCS device procedure, advanced age has been associated with higher risk of chronic lung disease, especially in the presence of previous history of smoking, and therefore, PFT can be an additional helpful prognostic tool in this patient population.[34,36] Presence of cardiogenic pulmonary edema may produce unreliable results especially in the setting of acute heart failure and therefore the test is not very helpful.

Hematologic consideration

Bleeding seems to be more frequent among frail and very old patients and plays an important role in the postprocedural phase of mechanical circulatory support.[37] Factors such as polypharmacy with drug–drug interaction, decreased renal/hepatic clearance, pharmacokinetic changes in the elderly, preexisting cerebrovascular condition and gastrointestinal bleeding and chronic anemia can all play a role in exacerbating bleeding, and it is important to pay more attention to anticoagulation aspect of MCS management in elderly and adopt a more individualized plan.

MALIGNANCIES

Advanced age is strongly associated with higher incidence of malignancies.[38] Patients with a history of recently treated or active cancer and a life expectancy of more than 2 years may be candidates for destination therapy if a multidisciplinary evaluation by oncologist, heart failure team, and patient and family will clear the postoperative path.

NUTRITIONAL STATUS

Malnutrition in the elderly is a challenging issue and is associated with increased mortality and morbidity, increased frailty, and reduced activities of daily living and quality of life in general.[39] Ability for a proper self-nourishment is a multifactorial issue affected by psychosocial status of the patient as well as mechanical considerations such as oral hygiene, partially or complete edentulous status, and poor gastrointestinal mucosal perfusion and nutrient absorption. Patients with evidence of severe malnutrition should have a proper dietary consultation, and their durable MCS should be postponed till their nutritional status is optimized. However, temporary MCS will allow to bridge this gap while waiting to improve the nutritional frailty.[34,39,40]

Palliative Care for the Elderly on Mechanical Circulatory Support

MCS devices have been shown to improve functional status and quality of life as well as survival. However, complications remain common and can have a significant impact on quality of life and even survival.[41–43] Furthermore, patients on MCS may face unanticipated challenges and complications, with operative course, which is less predictable and more complicated to prognosticate. Particularly, end-of-life experience for both patients and their families could be very challenging.[44,45] Hence, the palliative care team should be consulted throughout the course from decision-making period, preimplantation, and for the duration of therapy. They can guide difficult communications to establish goals of care and provide support to patient and family depending on their individual needs. Given the high morbidity and mortality with MCS, collaboration with palliative care is encouraged by the International Society for Heart and Lung Transplantation guidelines for MCS and considered a class IIa recommendation.[33] The Centers for Medicare and Medicaid Services and the Joint Commission further requires that a palliative care specialist be a part of the core multi-disciplinary MCS team.[46] Despite limited data on the efficacy of palliative care in patients with MCS, overall impressions of palliative care specialists are highly positive, with perceptions of improved patient and family experience and decreased burden on MCS team members.[47]

SUMMARY

Because MCS continues to advance with improving outcomes, careful patient selection among the elderly population will become increasingly important. Although mortality is higher in the elderly, carefully selected patients, MCS support can be valuable and lead to clinical recovery. The optimal use of MCS requires an individualized approach that is based on patient's comorbidities, the mechanism of a patient's disease, an understanding of the physiological effects of these devices, and the patient's potential clinical course. Age itself should not preclude patients from being candidates for MCS. Many institutions currently use arbitrarily selected age thresholds for MCS use, which precludes many elderly patients with minimal comorbidities from receiving MCS. The ability to select elderly patients who are most likely to benefit from MCS remains uncertain and warrants systematic study. Future studies will be needed to develop risk stratification tools to define those elderly patients for whom support is futile and those who will benefit the most from MCS.

CLINICS CARE POINTS

- Age is an independent risk factor for mortality in patients supported with MCS devices.
- Impella unloads the LV directly, leading to increase in cardiac output, a decrease in the LVEDP and decreasing myocardial oxygen consumption.
- VA-ECMO increases global systemic perfusion and mean arterial pressure, but it causes increased LV afterload, increase in LVEDP and pulmonary artery wedge pressure.
- Palliative care physician as a part of MCS team improves patient and family experience and decreases burden on MCS team members.

FUNDING STATEMENT

Support was provided solely from institutional and departmental sources. There were no external sources of funding.

DECLARATION OF INTERESTS

The authors declare no competing financial disclosure and conflict of interests.

REFERENCES

1. Gibbon JH Jr. Application of a mechanical heart and lung apparatus to cardiac surgery. Minn Med 1954;37(3):171–85.
2. Burkhoff D, Sayer G, Doshi D, et al. Hemodynamics of Mechanical Circulatory Support. J Am Coll Cardiol 2015;66(23):2663–74.
3. Prevention. CfDCa. Life expectancy at birth, at 65 years of age, and at 75 years of age, by race and sex: United States, selected years 1900-2007. Available at: https://www.cdc.gov/nchs/data/hus/2010/022.pdf. Accessed September 21, 2022.
4. Nations TU. The 2022 Revision of World Population Prospects. Available at: https://population.un.org/wpp/. Accessed September 20, 2022.
5. Frea S, Pidello S, Bovolo V, et al. Prognostic incremental role of right ventricular function in acute decompensation of advanced chronic heart failure. Eur J Heart Fail 2016;18(5):564–72.
6. Estep JD, Vivo RP, Krim SR, et al. Echocardiographic evaluation of hemodynamics in patients with systolic heart failure supported by a continuous-flow LVAD. J Am Coll Cardiol 2014;64(12):1231–41.
7. Seyfarth M, Sibbing D, Bauer I, et al. A randomized clinical trial to evaluate the safety and efficacy of a percutaneous left ventricular assist device versus intra-aortic balloon pumping for treatment of cardiogenic shock caused by myocardial infarction. J Am Coll Cardiol 2008;52(19):1584–8.
8. Moazami N, Fukamachi K, Kobayashi M, et al. Axial and centrifugal continuous-flow rotary pumps: a translation from pump mechanics to clinical practice. J Heart Lung Transplant 2013;32(1):1–11.
9. Kern MJ, Aguirre FV, Tatineni S, et al. Enhanced coronary blood flow velocity during intraaortic balloon counterpulsation in critically ill patients. J Am Coll Cardiol 1993;21(2):359–68.
10. van Nunen LX, Noc M, Kapur NK, et al. Usefulness of intra-aortic balloon pump counterpulsation. Am J Cardiol 2016;117(3):469–76.
11. Burkhoff D, Cohen H, Brunckhorst C, et al. A randomized multicenter clinical study to evaluate the safety and efficacy of the TandemHeart percutaneous ventricular assist device versus conventional therapy with intraaortic balloon pumping for treatment of cardiogenic shock. Am Heart J 2006;152(3):469 e1-8.
12. Patel B, Diaz-Gomez JL, Ghanta RK, et al. Management of extracorporeal membrane oxygenation for postcardiotomy cardiogenic shock. Anesthesiology 2021; 135(3):497–507.
13. Fan E, Brodie D, Slutsky AS. Acute respiratory distress syndrome: advances in diagnosis and treatment. JAMA 2018;319(7):698–710.
14. Acute Respiratory Distress Syndrome N, Brower RG, Matthay MA, et al. Ventilation with lower tidal volumes as compared with traditional tidal volumes for acute lung injury and the acute respiratory distress syndrome. N Engl J Med 2000; 342(18):1301–8.

15. Peek GJ, Mugford M, Tiruvoipati R, et al. Efficacy and economic assessment of conventional ventilatory support versus extracorporeal membrane oxygenation for severe adult respiratory failure (CESAR): a multicentre randomised controlled trial. Lancet 2009;374(9698):1351–63.
16. Patel B, Chatterjee S, Davignon S, et al. Extracorporeal membrane oxygenation as rescue therapy for severe hypoxemic respiratory failure. J Thorac Dis 2019; 11(Suppl 14):S1688–97.
17. Pappalardo F, Pieri M, Greco T, et al. Predicting mortality risk in patients undergoing venovenous ECMO for ARDS due to influenza A (H1N1) pneumonia: the EC-MOnet score. Intensive Care Med 2013;39(2):275–81.
18. Schmidt M, Zogheib E, Roze H, et al. The PRESERVE mortality risk score and analysis of long-term outcomes after extracorporeal membrane oxygenation for severe acute respiratory distress syndrome. Intensive Care Med 2013;39(10): 1704–13.
19. Schmidt M, Bailey M, Sheldrake J, et al. Predicting survival after extracorporeal membrane oxygenation for severe acute respiratory failure. The Respiratory Extracorporeal Membrane Oxygenation Survival Prediction (RESP) score. Am J Respir Crit Care Med 2014;189(11):1374–82.
20. Mendiratta P, Tang X, Collins RT 2nd, et al. Extracorporeal membrane oxygenation for respiratory failure in the elderly: a review of the Extracorporeal Life Support Organization registry. ASAIO J 2014;60(4):385–90.
21. Deatrick KB, Mazzeffi MA, Galvagno SM Jr, et al. Outcomes of venovenous extracorporeal membrane oxygenation when stratified by age: how old is too old? ASAIO J 2020;66(8):946–51.
22. Barbaro RP, MacLaren G, Boonstra PS, et al. Extracorporeal membrane oxygenation support in COVID-19: an international cohort study of the Extracorporeal Life Support Organization registry. Lancet 2020;396(10257):1071–8.
23. Pranikoff T, Hirschl RB, Steimle CN, et al. Mortality is directly related to the duration of mechanical ventilation before the initiation of extracorporeal life support for severe respiratory failure. Crit Care Med 1997;25(1):28–32.
24. Vallabhajosyula S, Dewaswala N, Sundaragiri PR, et al. Cardiogenic shock complicating st-segment elevation myocardial infarction: an 18-year analysis of temporal trends, epidemiology, management, and outcomes. Shock 2022; 57(3):360–9.
25. Hanna A, Frangogiannis NG. The cell biological basis for primary unloading in acute myocardial infarction. Int J Cardiol 2019;293:45–7.
26. Schafer A, Werner N, Burkhoff D, et al. Influence of timing and predicted risk on mortality in impella-treated infarct-related cardiogenic shock patients. Front Cardiovasc Med 2020;7:74.
27. Bagnall NM, Faiz O, Darzi A, et al. What is the utility of preoperative frailty assessment for risk stratification in cardiac surgery? Interact Cardiovasc Thorac Surg 2013;17(2):398–402.
28. Joseph SM, Manghelli JL, Vader JM, et al. Prospective assessment of frailty using the fried criteria in patients undergoing left ventricular assist device therapy. Am J Cardiol 2017;120(8):1349–54.
29. Joshi A, Mancini R, Probst S, et al. Sarcopenia in cardiac surgery: dual X-ray absorptiometry study from the McGill frailty registry. Am Heart J 2021;239:52–8.
30. Heberton GA, Nassif M, Bierhals A, et al. Usefulness of psoas muscle area determined by computed tomography to predict mortality or prolonged length of hospital stay in patients undergoing left ventricular assist device implantation. Am J Cardiol 2016;118(9):1363–7.

31. Teigen LM, John R, Kuchnia AJ, et al. Preoperative pectoralis muscle quantity and attenuation by computed tomography are novel and powerful predictors of mortality after left ventricular assist device implantation. Circ Heart Fail 2017; 10(9). https://doi.org/10.1161/CIRCHEARTFAILURE.117.004069.

32. Soud M, Alahdab F, Ho G, et al. Usefulness of skeletal muscle area detected by computed tomography to predict mortality in patients undergoing transcatheter aortic valve replacement: a meta-analysis study. Int J Cardiovasc Imaging 2019;35(6):1141–7.

33. Feldman D, Pamboukian SV, Teuteberg JJ, et al. The 2013 international society for heart and lung transplantation guidelines for mechanical circulatory support: executive summary. J Heart Lung Transplant 2013;32(2):157–87.

34. Peura JL, Colvin-Adams M, Francis GS, et al. Recommendations for the use of mechanical circulatory support: device strategies and patient selection: a scientific statement from the American Heart Association. Circulation 2012;126(22): 2648–67.

35. Knoepke CE, Chaussee EL, Matlock DD, et al. Changes over time in patient stated values and treatment preferences regarding aggressive therapies: insights from the DECIDE-LVAD trial. Med Decis Making 2022;42(3):404–14.

36. Hess NR, Seese LM, Hickey GW, et al. The predictive value of preimplant pulmonary function testing in LVAD patients. J Card Surg 2021;36(1):105–10.

37. Goldstein DJ, Beauford RB. Left ventricular assist devices and bleeding: adding insult to injury. Ann Thorac Surg 2003;75(6 Suppl):S42–7.

38. Driver JA, Djousse L, Logroscino G, et al. Incidence of cardiovascular disease and cancer in advanced age: prospective cohort study. BMJ 2008;337:a2467.

39. Norman K, Hass U, Pirlich M. Malnutrition in older adults-recent advances and remaining challenges. Nutrients 2021;13(8). https://doi.org/10.3390/nu13082764.

40. Genev I, Yost G, Gregory M, et al. Improved nutrition status in patients with advanced heart failure implanted with a left ventricular assist device. Nutr Clin Pract 2019;34(3):444–9.

41. Rogers JG, Aaronson KD, Boyle AJ, et al. Continuous flow left ventricular assist device improves functional capacity and quality of life of advanced heart failure patients. J Am Coll Cardiol 2010;55(17):1826–34.

42. McIlvennan CK, Magid KH, Ambardekar AV, et al. Clinical outcomes after continuous-flow left ventricular assist device: a systematic review. Circ Heart Fail 2014;7(6):1003–13.

43. Kirklin JK, Pagani FD, Kormos RL, et al. Eighth annual INTERMACS report: special focus on framing the impact of adverse events. J Heart Lung Transplant 2017;36(10):1080–6.

44. McIlvennan CK, Jones J, Allen LA, et al. Bereaved caregiver perspectives on the end-of-life experience of patients with a left ventricular assist device. JAMA Intern Med 2016;176(4):534–9.

45. Swetz KM, Ottenberg AL, Freeman MR, et al. Palliative care and end-of-life issues in patients treated with left ventricular assist devices as destination therapy. Curr Heart Fail Rep 2011;8(3):212–8.

46. Services. CfMaM. Decision memo for ventricular assist devices for bridge-to-transplant and destination therapy (CAG-00432R). Available at: https://www.cms.gov/medicare-coverage-database/details/nca-decision-memo.aspx?NCAId=268. Accessed September 20, 2022.

47. Sagin A, Kirkpatrick JN, Pisani BA, et al. Emerging Collaboration Between Palliative Care Specialists and Mechanical Circulatory Support Teams: A Qualitative Study. J Pain Symptom Manage 2016;52(4):491–497.e1.

Liver Transplantation and the Elderly Candidate: Perioperative Considerations

Andrea De Gasperi, MD[a],*, Laura Petrò, MD[b,c],
Elisabetta Cerutti, MD[d,e]

KEYWORDS

- Liver transplantation • Elderly candidate • Frailty • Preoperative evaluation
- Cardiac assessment • General anesthesia • Hemodynamic instability

KEY POINTS

- Preoperative frailty assessment is becoming imperative across all surgical specialties to ease risk stratification and shared decision-making and improve outcomes.
- Frailty is now recognized in 15% to 50% of end-stage liver disease (ESLD) patients. A user-friendly assessment tool (Liver Frailty Index [LFI]) is now available. As a growing number of older patients suffering from ESLD will be recipients of liver transplant (LT) surgery, LT series will be composed of up to 25% of older frail recipients.
- Perioperative medicine in LT surgery is an ever-expanding multidisciplinary activity. It should be managed by anaesthesiologists as "pivotal perioperative physicians" working in a multidisciplinary team. Their main aim should be to "merge" the work of hepatologists, surgeons, the "dedicated" cardiologist, physiotherapists, and nutritionists to ease the entire perioperative period in short to become the "perioperative transplant physician."

Continued

INTRODUCTION

The number of older subjects in the population is growing worldwide. Besides wisdom, however, ageing bears a heavy burden of comorbidities and a greater risk of health problems.[1] Recent US vital statistics show that close to 10% of surgical patients are 65 years or older, surgery being a key to solve some of their health problems (ASA Headquarter, 2022, accessed in September 2022). According to the *World Population Ageing* 2013, the United Nations defined older people as those aged 60 years or more. Recently, the World Health Organization (WHO) defined older people

[a] Anestesia Rianimazione 2 (AR2), ASST GOM Niguarda, Milan, Italy; [b] ANRI1 – Emergency and Intensive Care, ASST Ospedale Giovanni XXIII, Bergamo, Italy; [c] ASST Papa Giovanni XXII, Piazza MSO 1, 24100 Bergamo, Italy; [d] Anestesia e Rianimazione dei Trapianti e Chirurgia Maggiore, Azienda Ospedaliero Universitaria delle Marche, Via Conca 71, 60020, Ancona, Italy; [e] Azienda Ospedaliero Universitaria "Ospedali Riuniti", Via Conca 71, 60020, Ancona, Italy
* Corresponding author. Viale Porta Vercellina 20 20123, Milan.
E-mail address: andrea.degasperi@ospedaleniguarda.it

Anesthesiology Clin 41 (2023) 595–611
https://doi.org/10.1016/j.anclin.2023.02.009
1932-2275/23/© 2023 Elsevier Inc. All rights reserved.
anesthesiology.theclinics.com

Continued

- No formal guidelines are available so far for the pre-LT assessment of the elderly candidate. The "anesthesiologist–perioperative physician" should address central nervous, cardiovascular, respiratory, renal systems conditions, and comorbidities associated with ESLD, more often represented in the elderly candidate. Functional assessment tests should be integrated in the LT evaluation.
- LT anesthesia in the elderly must be based on solid knowledge of the physiologic changes associated to ageing. Hemodynamic instability could be more common in the older surgical patients making a proactive anesthesia management key to reducing complications. Changes in pharmacokinetic and pharmacodynamic characteristics should drive pharmacologic strategies and drugs choices.

in developed countries those aged 65 years or more or—alternatively—older persons who have passed their median life expectancy at birth.[1] In the pragmatic Europeak Community (EU) document, *Ageing Europe*,[2] old people are those aged 65 years or more, *very old people* those aged 85 years or more. Whatever the definition, by 2030 close to one-fifth of the population in developed countries will be aged 65 years or older,[1–3] and according to US statistics, every year about 21% of the elderly will undergo some form of anesthesia and surgery.[1,3] Such an increase of older patients needing any form of surgery—transplant and cardiac surgeries included—mandates improvements both in perioperative care delivery and outcomes.

AGE, AGEING, AND FRAILTY

Ageing is often associated with *frailty*, a "multisystem syndrome" closely correlated with decreases in physical, mental, and functional reserves. It is a "cumulative biological decline of multiple organ systems," leading to greater vulnerability to stressors and adverse health outcomes.[4] According to Thillainadesan and colleagues,[4] the ageing process should be considered a continuum, closely correlated with the severity and spread of biological changes in organs and tissues of older persons: the greater the changes in organs and tissues, the more likely is the individual to be frail. In 2020, George and colleagues[5] explored the association between frailty and postoperative mortality in over 2.7 million surgical patients across nine surgical specialties at various risk, stratified by operative stress scores. The investigators reported an association between frailty and postoperative morbidity and mortality in low-, moderate-, and high-risk surgical procedures. Frail and very frail patients had an incidence of 5.6% to 13.6% and 0.9% to 4.1%, respectively, of postoperative morbidity and mortality. In this very large series, George and colleagues[5] documented 10% mortality for frail patients at 180 days even in low-stress procedures and in low-intensity specialties. The results showed by George and colleagues underline once again the role of frailty, beyond the surgical stress itself, in the final surgical outcomes.[5–9] Unfortunately, preoperative frailty assessment is not routinely performed even before major abdominal surgery, as is in liver transplant (LT) surgery. According to Anderson and Wick in the accompanying editorial, frailty assessment "seems to be considered only as an afterthought."[10] Therefore, preoperative frailty assessment is imperative across all surgical specialties, regardless of case-mix, to ease risk stratification and support decision-making.[5,10] It is even more important in patients undergoing LT. Age, accumulated comorbidities, and increased vulnerability due to the reduced physiologic reserve are the mainstays of the frailty profile[6] and are included in the surgically validated Risk Analysis Index.[8,9]

AGE, FRAILTY, AND SARCOPENIA IN END-STAGE LIVER DISEASE: THE CHALLENGE OF THE LIVER TRANSPLANT INDICATION
Age and Liver Transplantation

Bajaj and colleagues[11] stress that together with the ageing of the population, diseases predominantly found in younger patients are now increasingly reported in the elderly. Chronic liver disease (CLD) in various forms—cirrhosis, alcohol-related liver disease (ALD), nonalcoholic fatty liver disease (NAFLD), nonalcoholic steatohepatitis (NASH), metabolic syndrome, and autoimmune cholestatic disease—and with different severity are nowadays reported in close to 2 billion people worldwide. Liver cirrhosis was the seventh most common cause of mortality in people older than 60 years in 2015 (*WHO Ageing and Health, 2016*, reported by Bajaj and colleagues).[11] These growing numbers of older patients suffering from end-stage liver disease (ESLD) in the United States and EU are obviously likely to become potential candidates or recipients of LT surgery,[12–15] this trend being evident both in the EU countries (**Fig. 1** from WWW.ELTR.org, accessed in September 2022) and United States[13,14] (**Figs. 2** and **3**).

Frailty and Liver Transplantation

LT, pioneered in the early 1970s as a "last ditch" treatment, is now a standardized, consolidated surgical procedure, considered the only curative option for patients with ESLD both in acute and chronic conditions.[15] LT is a high-risk surgical procedure, with substantial medical and surgical cutting edges.[12–17] Besides the donor organ shortage, stringent selective criteria are mandatory, and recipient age has always been considered one of the criteria for LT. Independently of age, and despite the prevalence in older patients, frailty is now recognized in all forms of CLD including ESLD. It has been reported in 15% to 50% of the patients with ESLD[16] and in up to 25% of the LT candidates.[17–20] In ESLD, liver failure, combined with neuromuscular, endocrine, immune, and skeletal muscle dysfunctions promote frailty. The underlying mechanisms leading to frailty in liver disease are far from being well understood and area

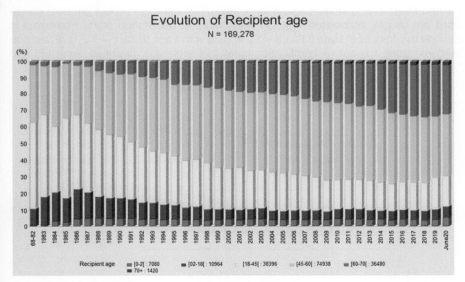

Fig. 1. Evolution of LT recipient age. (*From* ELTR registry from WWW ELTR.org, accessed in September 2022. No permission required.)

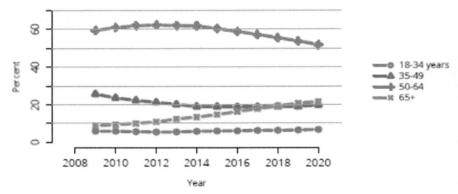

Fig. 2. Distribution of adults waiting for liver transplant by age. OPTN/SRTR 2020 Annual Data Report is not copyrighted. Readers are free to duplicate and use all or path of the information contained in this publication. Data are not copyrighted and may be used without permission if appropriate citation information is provided.

of active research.[16–18] In LT recipients, frailty *per se* has a significant impact on comorbidities, cognitive function and, in general, on overall complications and length of hospitalization.

Several prognostic tools have been studied and validated in the setting of frailty, such as Fried Frailty Index, short physical performance battery, 6-minute walk test (6MWT), and the Activities of Daily Living Scale.[18] To detect frailty in an ESLD patient in the easiest, most direct, and objective way, Lai and colleagues[19] proposed the Liver Frailty Index (LFI), a user-friendly objective tool consisting of three performance-based measures (grip strength, chair stands, and balance testing), specifically adapted to "measure" physical function in cirrhotic LT candidates. It has been validated in many studies and provides better risk prediction for waitlist mortality than the model for end-stage liver disease-sodium (MELD-Na).[19,20] Although robust physical conditions are usually associated with LFI less than 3.2, debilitation starts from what is defined the "pre-frail" state (LFI 3.2–4.5), ending with frank frailty (>4.5).[18] Lai and colleagues, using the net reclassification index in candidates classified using LFI and

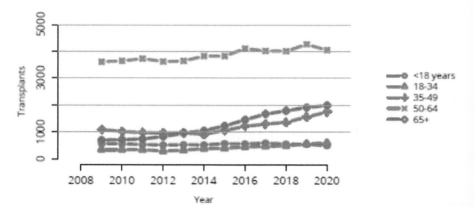

Fig. 3. Total liver transplant by age.

MELD-Na, were able to reclassify 19% of the LT candidates (16% of deaths/transplant waitlist de-listings and 3% of nondeaths/de-listings). The American Society of Transplantation strongly encourages the use of LFI in baseline and longitudinal assessment of LT candidates.[18] Using LFI, Haugen and colleagues[20] demonstrated frailty in one-third of older LT candidates, frailty being more common in older LT candidates than in younger ones (33.3% vs 21.6%). However, though a higher risk of waitlist mortality was independently associated with older age and frailty, frailty per se, regardless of the candidates' age, was associated with a twofold risk of waitlist mortality independent of the MELD-Na score.[20] This observation is further supported by the results in the 2020 Scientific Registry of Transplant Recipients report, where waitlist mortality analyzed by the age of candidates showed a sharp decrease in candidates over 65 since 2016 (**Figs. 4** and **5**). Frailty unfortunately was not included in the 2020 report but should be considered in the next reports due to the relevant impact it has on outcomes.[14,20].

Sarcopenia and Liver Transplantation

Sarcopenia, often reported together with frailty and indeed part of it, was initially considered as an age-related loss of muscle mass and function but is in fact a distinct entity and is now observed in all forms of CLD.[14,15,17,18,21] Although frailty is a clinical diagnosis including physical, mental, and psychosocial components, sarcopenia is a complex pathophysiologic change of muscles, with important functional consequence.[16–18,21] The skeletal muscle index (SMI) (height-normalized total abdominal muscle area at L3 level in abdominal computerized tomography [CT] scans) is the most widely used method to estimate total muscle mass.[17,18,21] Gender-specific cut-offs are still debated, as are the interpretations of the complex relationship between sarcopenia and outcomes in LT candidates.[21] Machine learning algorithms applied to the SMI and new MRI-based techniques are emerging as tools that are being used for more appropriate sarcopenia assessments. This said, it is well demonstrated that in case of low psoas thickness (<6.8 mm/m), the survival rate is lower and the hazard ratio for mortality is higher.[18] Frailty correlates with central sarcopenia; an appropriate nutritional assessment should be mandatory when managing the frail/sarcopenic LT candidate. In fact, up to 50% of the LT candidates have moderate, if not severe, malnutrition, unequivocally calling for both a dedicated pre-LT nutritional assessment and a tailored nutritional program.[21] Interestingly, according to Xu and

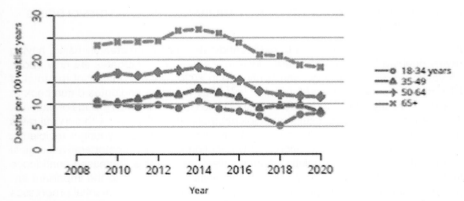

Fig. 4. Pretransplant mortality rate among adults wait-listed for liver transplant by age. (OPTN/SRTR 2020 Annual Data Report. HHS/HRSA.)

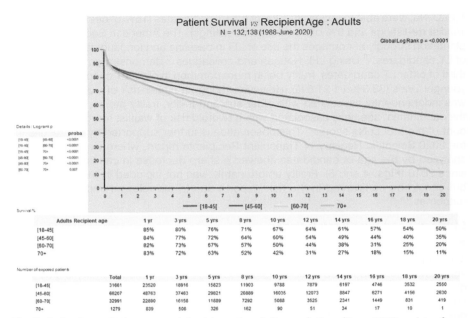

Fig. 5. Patients survival versus recipients' age in adult population. (*From* ELTR registry from WWW ELTR.org, accessed in September 2022. No permission required.)

colleagues, frailty is more common in patients with ALD, NAFLD, and "other etiologies" and was associated with waitlist mortality independent of cirrhosis etiology.[17,18,22] These findings should strongly support the need for frailty assessment across all CLD etiologies.[17,18,21] A preoperative assessment of elderly LT should undergo a mandatory formal and timely pre-LT assessment of frailty and sarcopenia, as well as obesity, often recorded in elderly frail/sarcopenic patients.[18] If the postoperative LT course threatens to be suboptimal (possibly leading to an undesirable outcome) for frail candidates,[7,8,17,18] the selection of suitable candidates for a tailored comprehensive prehabilitation should be considered.

LIVER TRANSPLANTATION IN THE OLDER CANDIDATE: WHAT ANESTHESIOLOGISTS SHOULD KNOW

As already noted, the numbers of older candidates for LT are steadily rising, having nearly doubled in the last 15 years; close to a quarter of candidates are now above 65 years of age, this having been confirmed in 2020, when a quarter of the total of LT patients were more than 65 years.[14,15,17,23] LT in older candidates dates back to late 1980 to early 1990, pioneered by Starzl[24] and Belzer[25] in small groups of patients. They reported very good results in recipients more than 60 years, with survival rates and incidence of perioperative complications similar to those in younger recipients; in fact, intraoperative complications, early rejection episodes, postoperative surgical complications, and opportunistic infections were comparable. Increased confidence in widening LT indications to the elderly was initially attributed to the important improvements in immunosuppressive therapy for the late 1980. Substantial progresses in modern immunosuppressive therapy, surgical, and medical care are now mainstays of current management of LT patients. According to the current American Association for the Study of Liver Disease (AASLD) 2013[26] and European Association for the Study of the Liver (EASL) 2018[27] guidelines, chronologic age is not by itself an absolute contraindication for LT: recipients aged 65 years but also 70 years (and beyond, up to 80!). Such patients now present in appreciable numbers in medium- and high-volume centers, with the same favorable short-to-medium term outcomes.[28]

These results, however, need to be appropriately discussed to optimize outcomes while maintaining equity and ethics in the LT indication. Tailored and more selective selection criteria ("stringent" according to Cottone and colleagues) must nowadays include biological age, assessed by frailty (LFI as an example) and should also explore functional reserve, sarcopenia, nutritional status, and comorbidities.[15,19,20] Older candidates are exposed, at least epidemiologically, to higher rates of cardiovascular (CV), respiratory, renal and neuropsychiatric comorbidities and related perioperative complications.[13,15,23,29] Two studies are relevant in this setting.[12,28] In the first one,[28] CV, respiratory, and neurologic complications had an age-related incremental increase, but unfortunately were not appropriately predicted by any of the available models. Perioperative mortality, major surgical, and medical postoperative complications, including infections, showed no difference between elderly and younger recipient groups, an effect possibly reflecting a high rate of exclusions during a "conservative" multidisciplinary pre-LT screening/selection.[28] Together with "the patient," for a comprehensive risk assessment, the "underlying liver pathology" plays a key role in LT in the elderly, hepatocellular carcinoma (HCC) and NASH being nowadays among the most common indications for LT.[12,15,23] In the second recent meta-analysis on LT in patients aged over 65 years,[12] early survival was substantially affected by the underlying liver pathology. The study, while confirming age more than 65 years as an independent prognostic factor for graft loss and mortality, clearly documented an indisputable difference in transplant survival according to the LT indication. Although mortality in HCC candidates did not differ between elderly and younger patients, survival was lower in older patients with ALD. Age might in fact have a lower impact in HCC recipients, often physically fit or "robust," whereas ALD is not infrequently associated (26%) with frailty, sarcopenia, and malnutrition and age-related comorbidities.[29] As an appropriate indication to LT is the game changer for older candidates, anesthesiologists, as important members of the pre-LT assessment team, should be aware of these problems when clearing for LT. Of course, appropriate donor–recipient matching is mandatory for the entire process to achieve the best results and avoid futile procedures.[13,30]

LIVER TRANSPLANTATION AND THE ELDERLY CANDIDATE: ANESTHESIOLOGIST POINT OF VIEW

No formal guidelines are available so far for pre-LT assessment of the elderly candidate.[13,15,23] As appropriately addressed by Akhtar,[13] age and CLD-related changes can affect the physiologic profile in different ways. The "anesthesiologist–perioperative physician" comprehensively assessing the elderly LT candidate must take an account of central nervous system (CNS), CV, and respiratory and renal system conditions.[13,27,28] Comorbidities not necessarily associated with ESLD, such as obesity, coronary artery disease (CAD), diabetes mellitus (DM), chronic obstructive pulmonary disease (COPD), or chronic renal failure are more often reported in the elderly and may affect the perioperative period and—more important—may even worsen after LT. Their impact on medium- and long-term outcomes, in the light of recent study results, calls for further large, more granular multicenter studies.[30,31] The most recent AASLD update to guide evaluation in adult LT candidates,[32] states that *"in the absence of significant comorbidities, older recipient age (>70 years) is not a contraindication to LT"* (grade 2-B). Relevant for the anesthesiologists is several points (6, 7, 9 to 14, 19, 23) that recommend, definition of the cardiac, pulmonary, and renal profiles, together with complete nutritional and infectious disease assessment (the last two subjects are graded 1-A).

NEUROLOGIC AND NEUROPSYCHIATRIC ASSESSMENT

Neurologic screening should be performed in every LT candidate.[13] Neurologic complications (mainly central, but also peripheral) are among the main causes of unfavorable outcomes in elderly recipients.[33–35] A thorough clinical and neurologic assessment is warranted to rule in/rule out and/or differentiate neurologic disorders. It should include risk factors and age-related comorbidities and a neuropsychiatric assessment. Among others, cerebral small vessel disease, a common neurologic condition in older patients, could become a target of pre-LT screening to establish whether it might influence postoperative outcomes.[34] Cognitive dysfunction, often considered age-related and associated with disruption of brain connectivity,[36,37] should be differentiated from diseases secondary to medical comorbidities (eg, DM or vascular pathologies).[33] These can include (1) cerebrovascular diseases, stroke/transient ischemic attack and the sleep apnea syndrome, frequently reported in NASH/NAFLD patients, and substantial risk factor for stroke, stroke recurrence, and poor functional recovery[38,39]; (2) hepatic encephalopathy (HE), a complex, CLD-CNS dysfunction, manifesting as a wide spectrum of neurologic and psychiatric deficits. HE can be precipitated by acute or chronic "hits" which can lead to increase in an influx of neurotoxins (ammonia among others) not matched by adequate clearance of toxins, mediators, and cytokines[33,40,41]; (3) neurodegenerative diseases involving progressive loss of selectively vulnerable populations of neurons, different from the selective "static" neuronal loss associated with metabolic or toxic disorders[42]; and (4) infectious diseases.[33]

THE CARDIOVASCULAR PROFILE OF THE OLDER CANDIDATE AND ITS ASSESSMENT: STILL WAITING FOR A CONSENSUS

Ageing and age-related diseases, as documented in the most recent reports from both the United States[43] and EU,[44] are unequivocally associated with a high prevalence of "extended" and cumulative CV risk factors/diseases (age, CAD, hypertension, smoking, DM, metabolic syndrome, obesity, NASH) and polytherapy.[45] According to Alexander and colleagues,[46] three or more CV risk factors provide high sensitivity and specificity for detecting severe asymptomatic CAD in LT candidates, thus supporting older guidelines.[26,27,47] This risk profile is increasingly reported among elderly LT candidates, with a higher prevalence of (1) asymptomatic CAD (reported in up to 25% of older LT recipients)[48,49]; (2) heart failure (HF); (3) arrhythmias (among others, atrial fibrillation, documented in 1%–6% of the candidates, frequently reported among the postoperative cardiac complications and able to negatively impact the early postoperative course) and prolonged corrected QT (QTc) interval, both justifying the basal electrocardiogram (EKG); (4) valvular heart disease (well tolerated if mild to moderate, but becoming a contraindication in case of severe forms and need to be discussed in multidisciplinary meetings pre-LT for possible correction)[50]; (5) cirrhotic cardiomyopathy, recently redefined and readdressed with a new definition and a new clinical and echocardiographic assessment.[51,52] CV morbidity and mortality (30-day risk of major adverse cardiac events [MACEs], mainly CV death, myocardial infarction, and stroke) can be high and are mainly determined by two factors, the patient-related risk(s), frailty included, and the high-risk surgical procedure (MACEs > 5% for LT surgery).[48,53] A detailed preoperative assessment and careful selection of the candidate are pivotal to (1) reduce the perioperative risk(s), by identifying "active" cardiac conditions which can impact intraoperative and postoperative outcomes[49,53] and (2) decide in a multidisciplinary discussion if these active condition(s) should undergo correction before LT to improve the LT outcome.[53] As an example, in AASLD 2022 update states that "cardiac revascularization should be considered in LT candidates with significant coronary artery stenosis prior to transplant"(Grade 2-C).[32]

First formally addressed in 2012,[47] a formal CV risk assessment for LT surgery was proposed by American Heart Association/American College of Cardiology guidelines in 2013[26] and EASL in 2016,[27] then comprehensively reproposed by Barman and colleagues[50] and very recently included and graded by AASLD in the short 2022 update.[32] Two main targets of the CV assessment of an LT candidate are (even more strongly recommended for an older patient) to (1) establish whether a patient can be expected to survive the operation and the immediate postoperative period and (2) understand if LT should be considered inappropriate or even futile in an older candidate with severe cardiopulmonary disease/extreme frailty because of the chronic donor organs shortage.[31,49,54–57] The wide heterogeneity in cardiac risk screening strategies very recently documented in a US survey[54] (the same is in European Union),[55] together with the variable CV disease prevalence in LT candidates worldwide, shows once again, the importance of developing and validating a modern, evidence-based, CV risk prediction model.[47,54–57]

A few more points deserve attention (1) the importance of a "dedicated" cardiologist to be involved in the multidisciplinary pre-LT evaluation team[54,57] and (2) the importance of up-to-date and finalized pre-LT echocardiographic study in the prognostication and risk stratification of transplant candidates.[50,52–60] For special considerations on "older" guidelines (concerns about stress tests in general and stress echocardiography in ESLD setting in particular)[50,51,54–57] and for up-to-date insights, we suggest the recent comprehensive reviews.[50,51,54–60]

According to Levy and colleagues,[56] particular attention should focus on echocardiography with tissue Doppler imaging and strain imaging. Anatomic and functional consequences of CAD in LT candidates should become part of the risk stratification tool,[49,53] focusing the attention on an anatomical-based approach to CAD risk stratification. As an example, coronary computed tomography angiography (CCTA), championed by the Asiatic centers but much less used in United States and Europe, should be strongly considered in view of its excellent negative predictive value (97.5%) for post-LT MI.[61] Should CCTA be abnormal or contraindicated, invasive coronary artery angiography—the gold standard—should be performed.[31,50,53,57] Fine-tuning the noninvasive anatomical imaging could be a further step forward.[62.]

Portopulmonary hypertension (PoPH), even if rare (2%–5%), should be ruled out in older LT candidates by routine echocardiography; right heart cardiac catheterization is indicated in a patient with estimated right ventricular systolic pressure ≥45 mm Hg or pulmonary artery systolic pressure ≥45 mm Hg.[31,63] PoPH is classified according to mean Pulmonary artery pressure (mPAP) at right heart catheterization as mild (25–35 mm Hg), moderate (35–45 mm Hg), or severe (>45 mm Hg). According to the most recent guidelines,[64,65] patients with moderate PoPH (mPAPs > 35 but less than 50 mm Hg) should be temporarily delisted, referred to a PoPH specialist, treated with dedicated cardiac or pulmonary consultation for vasodilator therapy,[32,64,65] and reassessed for LT if they respond to medical therapy (mPAP ≤35 mm Hg).[32,64,65] Moderate PoPH with preserved right ventricular function not responsive to medical treatment is a relative contraindication to LT,[66] while persistent severe PoPH with right HF, not responsive to medical therapies, is an absolute contraindication, as the risk of right ventricular failure and post-LT mortality is extremely high.[63–66]

Even though pre-LT cardiac assessment is worldwide considered a priority,[50,55,56,67,68] it is still defined "a challenge."[67] Many questions, particularly *Who* should be screened for CAD, *Which* screening modality should be used, and *When* should the asymptomatic LT candidate repeat cardiac evaluation, do await consistent, evidence-based recommendations.[49,50,54,66]

THE FUNCTIONAL ASSESSMENT IN THE OLDER CANDIDATE: THE WAY TO ENHANCED RECOVERY AFTER SURGERY

A recent document dealing with enhanced recovery after surgery (ERAS), after LT,[69,70] states that functional assessment has a major role in this setting.[69–71] The DASI Score (Duke Activity Status Index) is a more objective version of the "old" metabolic equivalent of tasks score and is based on a well-defined questionnaire[72,73]; the cardiopulmonary exercise testing (CPET)[74] and the 6MWT[75] have a consolidated role in preoperative risk stratification and in predicting adverse cardiac and respiratory events after major noncardiac surgeries, including LT.[73–75] CPET and 6MWT have recently been defined as "reliable tests" to provide information on the cardiopulmonary endurance and the burden of physical deconditioning.[74,75] CPET, perhaps the most accurate marker of cardiopulmonary fitness, has two main limitations: the specialized equipment/personnel required and conducting it in critically ill patients. The 6MWT is a simpler and more user-friendly tool and can provide a viable alternative option; however, data to support the 6MWT for risk stratification in the LT setting, in general and in ERAS protocols in particular, are lacking so far.[69] Tracking the physiologic progress in functional capacity during tailored prehabilitation training programs should enable physicians to understand whether or not the frail candidates will tolerate the physiologic stress imposed by the LT, optimizing the entire LT program and improving outcomes.[69]

THE PERIOPERATIVE PERIOD OF LIVER TRANSPLANTATION: FACING A MARATHON!

The safety of modern anesthesia management relies, among others factors, on attention to the changes induced by surgery on the patient's physiologic profile and appropriate intraoperative monitoring strategy.[76] Anesthesia in the elderly candidates should be based on solid knowledge of the physiologic changes associated to ageing and response to various phases of surgery.[13,37,77]

Intraoperative hypotension, a feared and increasingly reported complication during anesthesia, is more common in the elderly surgical patients and a major problem during LT.[76,78–81]: Changes in pharmacokinet / pharmacodynamic (PK/PD) characteristics should drive pharmacologic strategies and drugs choices.[13,37,77] The extensive, tailored, thorough preoperative assessment, "able to clear a patient for a surgical procedure close to running a marathon"[82] is more than justified by what every LT anesthesiologist experiences during the various phases of the LT.[78–81] The patient may have to tolerate periods (minutes to hours) of critical and multifactorial hemodynamic instability the result, among others, of decreased preload, decreased systemic vascular resistance, impaired myocardial performance, or a combination of the three.[80] The many components of hemodynamic instability during LT include severe hypotension, tachycardia/tachyarrhythmias, malignant ventricular tachyarrhythmias, metabolic acidosis, major acute volume shifts (acute hemorrhage, extreme anemia, massive transfusion, and sudden and severe reduction of venous return), prolonged and resistant vasoplegia after reperfusion of the graft (10%–80% of the cases), acute right or left ventricular overload, dynamic left ventricular outflow obstruction, cardiac tamponade, intracardiac thrombosis/pulmonary embolisms (2%–6%), and cardiac arrest (3.7%).[81]

Surgical bleeding or "coagulopathy" in LT patients is much better understood and managed in the last 15 years. Major innovations and advances in surgical techniques have led to a more informed perioperative management of transfusion[83–85] and fluid administration policies.[86,87] The presence of specifically trained ("designated") anesthesiology teams and a proactive perioperative management have led to, reduced blood/blood components use, less fluid overload, and improved postoperative outcomes.[88] Age per se does not seem to affect surgical time but is among the factors able to significantly affect blood losses and perioperative complications.[89,90] As recently reported by Mousa and colleagues[90] in a large single-center study on the elderly LT recipients, the risk of death was not significantly higher than among recipients younger than 60 years. Among elderly recipients, greater packed red blood cell requirement and longer warm ischemia time were significantly associated with decreased survival.[90] Mousa and colleagues[90] introduced the concept of "restoration of life expectation" provided by the LT procedure on lifespan relative to patients' ages. As already mentioned, a thorough preoperative cardiac assessment is more than justified because of (1) the rate of perioperative adverse CV events (close to 40% of early total post-LT mortality); (2) MACEs more frequent among elderly patients suffering for NASH, DM, hypertension, and COPD.[15] Older age together with DM and COPD were associated with higher rate of cardiac arrest.[81] As appropriately underlined by Cottone and colleagues,[15] a "selection bias" introduced by the "mandatory" strict candidate selection might have affected the intraoperative complication rate, in the real world perhaps even higher than reported.

For the early postoperative period, ICU length of stay shows great variability among LT centers, particularly in case of older and frail recipients. Fast-tracks protocols have long been proposed with outstanding results supported by modern intraoperative management, early extubation,[78–80] and ERAS protocols.[70,71] Good results after LT were reported quite recently with septuagenarian recipients. These elderly patients did not differ from younger patients in surgical complications, need for mechanical ventilation, length of ICU and hospital stays, and readmission after LT.[91] However, a very recent Australian survey reported a higher short- and long-term mortality, longer ICU stay, prolonged artificial ventilation in frail surgical patients admitted to ICU.[92] Therefore, appropriate, candidate selection and tailored comprehensive prehabilitation programs are key to run an LT program in the elderly, whose main aim should be to optimize resources—scarce by definition——to "expand lifespan expectations."[90]

Beside the comprehensive and up to date "standard" assessment, we have tried to address—frailty assessment included—major anatomical, pathophysiologic, and surgical issues associated with intraoperative and postoperative complications and adverse events (bleeding, transfusion, ischemia times, among others). However, every transplant center, from its own results, should aim, as far as possible, to avoid every preventable adverse events,[90–92] implementing on modifiable variables every measure able to have a positive impact on grafts and patients outcomes.

SUMMARY

The CV metabolic and respiratory stress imposed by the LT surgery to the recipients[79–82] has recently been described by Hogan "akin to running a marathon."[83] To "challenge the marathon," candidates, frail because of ESLD but even more frail because older, should be fully assessed, and when cleared for LT, "intensively" trained. The comprehensive preoperative assessment, including frailty evaluation, should be followed by tailored, dynamic pre-habilitation, and nutritional programs. Infections and infection-related risk factors should be assessed, ruled out or in any case solved. Since the late 1980, elderly candidates have been more and more confidently cleared for LT; older recipients (65 years and older) now account for up to 25% in most of the United States, EU, and Asian series, numbers that are likely to increase in the very near future. Results are constantly improving and according to the most recent data able to restore the lifespan expectation of the elderly: the challenge cannot be refused!

CLINICS CARE POINTS

- Older candidates/recipients are nowadays the rule and not the exception in liver transplant (LT) programs
- Older end-stage liver disease patients are often frail; anesthesiologists should become acquainted with such a peculiar patient, having a solid knowledge of the elderly physiologic profile for a wise management of the perioperative period.
- Preoperative LT evaluation, together with a preoperative "elderly–oriented" pathway, should mandatorily include the frailty assessment using Liver Frailty Index and a functional assessment, this latter extremely useful to explore the cardiovascular and the neurologic profiles and to orient the need for prehabilitation.
- Anesthesiologists involved in LT surgery should become the "true" perioperative transplant physicians, merging the multidisciplinary preoperative work done by surgeons, hepatologists, and cardiologist(s) to ease the perioperative period.
- Having such an active part in the older candidates selection, anesthesiologists will play a relevant role in increasing the already good early- and medium-term LT results, avoiding futile procedures while (hopefully) expanding recipients' expanding lifespan expectations.

CONFLICTS OF INTEREST

None.

ACKNOWLEDGEMENTS

To Ernestina Mazza, MD, and Stefano Skurzak, MD, for the acute and fruitful suggestions. To Gloria Innocenti, ASST GOM Niguarda Librarian. To Judith Baggott for the English editing.

REFERENCES

1. Ageing and health - World Health Organization. Available at: https://www.who.int/news-room/fact-sheets/detail/ageing-and-health. Accessed Sept 2022.
2. Ageing Europe 2019 - looking at the lives of older people in the EU. European Union; 2019.
3. Perioperative Medicine - UCSF Dept of Anesthesia. Available at: https://anesthesia.ucsf.edu/research-group/perioperative-medicine.
4. Thillainadesan J, Scott IA, Le Couteur DG. Frailty, a multisystem ageing syndrome. Age Ageing 2020;49:758–63.

5. George EL, Hall DE, Youk A, et al. Association between patient frailty and post-operative mortality across multiple noncardiac surgical specialties. JAMA Surg 2021;156:e205152.

6. Rockwood K, Song X, MacKnight C, et al. A global clinical measure of fitness and frailty in elderly people. CMAJ (Can Med Assoc J) 2005;173(5):489–95.

7. Hall DE, Arya S, Schmid KK, et al. Development and initial validation of the risk analysis index for measuring frailty in surgical populations. JAMA Surg 2017; 152(2):175–82.

8. Arya S, Varley P, Youk A, et al. Recalibration and external validation of the risk analysis index: a surgical frailty assessment tool. Ann Surg 2019. https://doi.org/10.1097/SLA0000000000003276.

9. Varley PR, Borrebach JD, Arya S, et al. Clinical utility of the risk analysis index as a prospective frailty screening tool within a multi-practice, multi-hospital integrated healthcare system. Ann Surg 2020. https://doi.org/10.1097/SLA0000000000003808.

10. Anderson D. Wick EC frailty and postoperative morbidity and mortality—here, there, and everywhere. JAMA Surg 2021;156(1):e205153.

11. Bajaj S, Gentili A, Wade JB, et al. Specific challenges in geriatric cirrhosis and hepatic encephalopathy. Clin Gastroenterol Hepatol 2022;20:S20–9.

12. Gómez-Gavara C, Lim C, Adam R, et al. The impact of advanced patient age in liver transplantation: a European liver transplant registry propensity-score matching study. HBP 2022;24:974–85.

13. Aktar S. Preoperative evaluation of geriatric patients undergoing liver transplantation. Curr Op Crit Care 2022;35:96–104.

14. Kwong AJ, Ebel NH, Kim WR, et al. OPTN/SRTR 2020 annual data report. SRTR (as accessed Sept 18) also published in. Am J Transplant 2022;22(Suppl 2): 204–309.

15. Cottone C, Pena Polanco NA, Bhamidimarri KR. Transplant of elderly patients: is there an upper age cutoff? Clin Liver Dis 2021;25:209–27.

16. Laube R, Wang H, Park L, et al. Frailty in advanced liver disease. Liver Int 2018; 38:2117–28.

17. Schaenman J, Goldwaterb D, Malinisc M. An interdisciplinary approach to the older transplant patient: strategies for improving clinical outcomes. Curr Opin Organ Transplant 2019;24:504–10.

18. Liapakis AM, Morris E, Emre S. Frailty in liver transplantation: a comprehensive review. Hepatology Forum 2021;2:80–8.

19. Lai JC, Covinsky KEMD, Charles E, et al. The liver frailty index improves mortality prediction of the subjective clinician assessment in patients with cirrhosis. Am J Gastroenterol 2018;113:235–42.

20. Haugen CE, McAdamms DeMarco, Holsher CM, et al. Multicenter study of age, frailty, and waitlist mortality among liver transplant candidates. Ann Surg 2020; 271:1132–6.

21. Saiman Y, Serper M. Frailty and Sarcopenia in patients pre- and post-liver transplant. Clin Liver Dis 2021;25:35–51.

22. Xu CQ, Mohamad Y, Kappus ME, et al. The relationship between frailty and cirrhosis etiology: from the functional assessment in liver transplantation (FrAILT) study. Liver Int 2021;41:2467–73.

23. Dolnikov S, Adam R, Cherqui D, et al. Liver transplantation in elderly patients: what do we know at the beginning of 2020? Surg Today 2020;50:533–9.

24. Starzl TE, Todo S, Gordon R, et al. Liver transplantation in older patients. N Engl J Med 1987;316:484–5.

25. Pirsch JD, Kalayoglu M, D'Alessando M, et al. Orthotopic liver transplantation in patients 60 years of age and older. Transplantation 1991;51:431–3.

26. Martin P, DiMartini A, Feng S, et al. Evaluation for liver transplantation in adults: 2013 practice guideline by the American association for the study of liver diseases and the American society of transplantation. Hepatology 2014;59: 1144–65 (Updated march 15 2022 accessed at Available at: https://www.guidelinecentral.com/guideline/10759/AASLD).

27. EASL clinical practice guidelines: liver transplantation. J Hepatol 2016;64: 433–85.

28. Gómez Gavara C, Esposito F, Gurusamy K, et al. Liver transplantation in elderly patients: a systematic review and first meta-analysis. HPB 2019;21:14–25.

29. Lai JC, Dodge JL, McCulloch CE, et al. Frailty and the burden of concurrent and incident disability in patients with cirrhosis: a prospective cohort study. Hepatol Commun 2020;4:126–33.

30. Krissa M, Biggins SW. Evaluation and selection of the liver transplant candidate: updates on a dynamic and evolving process. Curr Opin Organ Transplant 2021; 26:52–61.

31. Lai JC. Defining the threshold for too sick for transplant. Curr Opin Organ Transplant 2016;21:127–32.

32. AASLD Update March 15 22. Available at: https://www.guidelinecentral.com/guideline/10759/DOI 10.1002/hep.26972.

33. Feltracco P, Cagnin A, Carollo C, et al. Neurological disorders in liver transplant candidates: pathophysiology and clinical assessment. Transplant Rev 2017;31: 193–206.

34. Avorio F, Sparacia G, Russeli G, et al. Neurological screening in elderly liver transplantation candidates: a single center experience. Neurol Int 2022;14: 245–55.

35. Zivkovic SA. Neurologic complications after liver transplantation. World J Hepatol 2013;5:409–16.

36. Edde M, Leroux G, Altena E, et al. Functional brain connectivity changes across the human lifespan: from fetal development to old age. J Neurosci Res 2021;99: 236–62.

37. Akhtar S. Neurological aging and pharmacological management of geriatric patients. Curr Anesthesiol Rep 2021;11:381–6.

38. Baillieul S, Dekkers M, Brill AK, et al. Sleep apnoea and ischaemic stroke: current knowledge and future directions. Lancet Neurol 2022;21:78–88.

39. Parikh MP, Gupta NM, McCullough AJ. Obstructive Sleep Apnea and the Liver. Clin Liver Dis 2019;23:363–82.

40. Wjidicks ECM. Hepatic encephalopathy. N Engl J Med 2016;375:1660–70.

41. Kumar G, Taneja A, Kandiah PA. Brain and the liver: cerebral edema, hepatic encephalopathy and beyond. In: Nanchal R, Subramanian R, editors. Hepatic critical care. Springer; 2018. p. 83–108.

42. Dugger B, Dickson DW. Pathology of neurodegenerative diseases. Cold Spring Harb Perspect Biol 2016;9:a028035.

43. Tsao CW, Aday AW, Zaid I, et al. Heart disease and stroke statistics—2022 update: a report from the american heart association. heart disease and stroke statistics—2022 update: a report from the American Heart Association. Circulation 2022;145:e153–639.

44. Task Force for. cardiovascular disease prevention in clinical practice with representatives of the European Society of Cardiology and 12 medical societies. 2021

ESC Guidelines on cardiovascular disease prevention in clinical practice. Eur Heart J 2021;42(34):3227–327.

45. Mohebali D, Anagnostopoulos AM, Estrada-Roman A, et al. Cardiovascular risk assessment in renal and liver transplant candidates: a multidisciplinary institutional standardized approach. Cardiol Rev 2019;27:286–92.

46. Alexander S, Teshome M, Patel H, et al. The diagnostic and prognostic utility of risk factors defined by the AHA/ACCF on the evaluation of cardiac disease in liver transplantation candidates. BMC Cardiovasc Disord 2019;19:102.

47. Lentine KL, Costa SP, Weir MR, et al. Cardiac disease evaluation and management among kidney and liver transplantation candidates: a scientific statement from the American Heart Association and the American College of Cardiology Foundation. J Am Coll Cardiol 2012;60:434–80.

48. Xiao J, Yong JN, Ng CH, et al. A meta-analysis and systematic review on the global prevalence, risk factors, and outcomes of coronary artery disease in liver transplantation recipients. Liver Transplant 2022;28:689–99.

49. Izzy M, VanWagner L. Coronary artery disease assessment during evaluation for liver transplantation: how much does it matter? Liver Transpl 2022;28:556–7.

50. Barman PM, VanWagner LB. Cardiac risk assessment in liver transplant candidates: current controversies and future directions. Hepatology 2021;73:2564–76.

51. Izzy M, VanWagner LB, Lin G, et al. Redefining cirrhotic cardiomyopathy for the modern era. Hepatology 2020;71:334–45.

52. Kleb C, Faisal MS, Quintini C, et al. C Factors predicting futility of liver transplant in elderly recipients: A single-center experience. World J Transplant 2021;11:421–31.

53. ESC Guidelines on cardiovascular assessment and management of patients undergoing non-cardiac surgery. Developed by the task force for cardiovascular assessment and management of patients undergoing non-cardiac surgery of the European Society of Cardiology (ESC). Endorsed by the European Society of Anaesthesiology and Intensive Care (ESAIC). Eur Heart J 2022;28:501–4.

54. Barman PM, Chadha RM, VanWagner LB. Cardiac risk assessment in liver transplant candidates: a survey of national practice patterns. Liver Transpl 2022;28:501–4.

55. DeGasperi A, Spagnolin G, Ornaghi M, et al. Preoperative cardiac assessment in liver transplant candidates. Best Pract Res Clin Anesth 2020;34:51–68.

56. Levy PE, Khan SS, VanWagner L. Cardiac evaluation of the kidney or liver transplant candidate. Curr Opin Organ Transplant 2021;26:77–84.

57. Truby LK, Mentz RJ, Agarwal R. Cardiovascular risk stratification in the noncardiac solid organ transplant candidate. Curr Opin Organ Transplant 2022;27:22–8.

58. Lim WH, Chew NWS, Queck J, et al. Echocardiographic assessment of cardiovascular function and clinical outcomes in liver transplant recipients. Clin Transplant 2022. https://doi.org/10.1111/ctr.14793.

59. Bushyhead D, Kirkpatrick JN, Goldberg D. Pretransplant echocardiographic parameters as markers of posttransplant outcomes in liver transplant recipients. Liver Transpl 2016;22:316–23.

60. Moon YJ, Kim JW, Bang YS, et al. Prediction of all-cause mortality after liver transplantation using left ventricular systolic and diastolic function assessment. PLoS One 2019;14:0209100.

61. Moon Y-J, Kwon H-M, Jung K-W, et al. Risk stratification of myocardial injury after liver transplantation in patients with computed tomographic coronary angiography-diagnosed coronary artery disease. Am J Transplant 2019;19:2053–66.

62. DeGasperi A, Zorzi A. Cardiac evaluation before liver transplantation: a step forward? J Hepatol 2021. https://doi.org/10.1016/j.jhep.2021.01.008.
63. Raevens S, Colle I, Reyntjens K, et al. Echocardiography for the detection of portopulmonary hypertension in liver transplant candidates: an analysis of cutoff values. Liver Transpl 2013;19:602–10.
64. Krowka MJ, Fallon MB, Kawut SM, et al. International liver transplant society practice guidelines: diagnosis and management of hepatopulmonary syndrome and portopulmonary hypertension. Transplantation 2016;100:1440–52.
65. Cartin Ceba R, Krowka MJ. Pulmonary complications of portal hypertension. Clin Liver Dis 2019;23:683–711.
66. VanWagner LB, Harinstein ME, Runo JR, et al. Multidisciplinary approach to cardiac and pulmonary vascular disease risk assessment in liver transplantation: an evaluation of the evidence and consensus recommendations. Am J Transplant 2018;18:30–42.
67. Sandal S, Chen T, Cantarovich M. The challenges with the cardiac evaluation of liver and kidney transplant candidates. Transplantation 2020;104:251–8.
68. Bonu M, Mavrogeni S, Capelios CJ, et al. Preoperative evaluation of coronary artery disease in liver transplant candidates: many unanswered questions in clinical practice. Diagnostics 2021;11:75.
69. Crespo G, Hessheimer AJ, Armstrong MJ. Which preoperative assessment modalities best identify patients who are suitable for enhanced recovery after liver transplantation? – A systematic review of the literature and expert panel recommendations. Clin Transplant 2022;36(10):e14644.
70. Available at: https://ERAS4OLT.org.
71. Brustia R, Monsel A, Skurzak S, et al. Guidelines for perioperative care for liver transplantation: enhanced recovery after surgery (ERAS) society recommendations. Transplantation 2022;106:552–61.
72. Wijeysundera D, Pearse RM, Schulman MA, et al. Assessment of functional capacity before major non-cardiac surgery: an international, prospective cohort study. Lancet 2018;391:2631–40.
73. Wijeysundera D, Beattie WS, Hillis GS, et al. Integration of the duke activity status Index into preoperative risk evaluation: a multicentre prospective cohort study. Br J Anaesth 2020;124:261–70.
74. Bernal W, Mateos RM, Lipcsey M, et al. Aerobic capacity during cardiopulmonary exercise testing and survival with and without liver transplantation for patients with chronic liver disease. Liver Transpl 2014;20:54–62.
75. Dang TNT, Ebadi M, Abraldes JG, et al. The 6-minute walk test distance predicts mortality in cirrhosis: a cohort of 694 patients awaiting liver Transplantation. Liver Transpl 2021;27:1490–2.
76. Brienza N, Biancofiore G, Cavaliere F, et al. Clinical guidelines for perioperative hemodynamic management of non cardiac surgical adult patients. Minerva Anestesiol 2019;85:1315–33.
77. Wahlen BM, DeGasperi A. Anesthetic concerns in advanced age undergoing emergency surgery. In: Latifi R, Catena F, Coccolini F, editors. Emergency General surgery in geriatrics. Springer nature Switzerland; 2021. p. 97–128.
78. Barjaktarevic I, Cotes Lopez R, Steadman R, et al. Perioperative consideration in Liver transplantation. Semin Respir Crit Care Med 2018;39:609e24.
79. Wagener G. Anesthesia for liver transplantation. Wolters Kluwer Health; 2019. UPTODATE. Literature review current through: Aug 2022. | This topic last updated: Jun 23, 2021.

80. Bezinover D, Muktar M, Wagener G, et al. Hemodynamic instability during liver transplantation in patients with end-stage liver disease: a consensus document from ILTS. LICAGE, and SATA 2021;105(10):2184–200.
81. Smith NK, Zerillo J, Kim SJ, et al. Intraoperative cardiac arrest during adult liver transplantation: incidence and risk factor analysis from 7 academic centers in the United States. Anesth Analg 2021;132:130–9.
82. Hogan BJ, Gonsalkorala E, Heneghan MA. Evaluation of coronary artery disease in potential liver transplant candidates. Liver Transpl 2017;23:386–95.
83. Tripodi A, Mannucci PM. The coagulopathy of chronic liver disease. N Engl J Med 2011;365:147–56.
84. Bezinover D, Dirkmann D, Findlay, et al. Perioperative coagulation management in liver transplant recipients. Transplantation 2018;102:578–92.
85. Pillai AA, Kriss M, Al-Adra DP, et al. Coagulopathy and hemostasis management in patients undergoing liver transplantation: Defining a dynamic spectrum across phases of care. Liver Transpl 2022;28:1651–63.
86. Carrier FM, Chassé M, Wang HT, et al. Restrictive fluid management strategies and outcomes in liver transplantation: a systematic review. Can J Anaesth 2020;67:109–27.
87. Carrier FM, Chassé M, Sylvestre MP, et al. Effects of intraoperative fluid balance during liver transplantation on postoperative acute kidney injury: an observational cohort study. Transplantation 2020;104:1419–28.
88. Hevesi ZG, Lopukhin SY, Mezrich JD, et al. Designated liver transplant anesthesia team reduces blood transfusion, need for mechanical ventilation, and duration of intensive care. Liver Transpl 2009;15:460–5.
89. Eghbal MH, Samadi K, Khosravi MB, et al. The impact of preoperative variables on intraoperative blood loss and transfusion requirements during orthotopic liver transplant. Experiment Clin Transplant 2019;17:507–12.
90. Mousa OY, Nguyen JH, Ma Y, et al. Evolving role of liver transplantation in elderly recipients. Liver Transplant 2019;25:1363–74.
91. Aduen JF, Sujay B, Dickson RC, et al. Outcomes after liver transplant in patients aged 70 years or older compared with those younger than 60 years. Mayo Clin Proc 2009;84:973–8.
92. Chan R, Ueno R, Afroz A, et al. Association between frailty and clinical outcomes in surgical patients admitted to intensive care units: a systematic review and meta-analysis. Br J Anaesth 2021. https://doi.org/10.1016/j.bja.2021.11.018.

Perioperative Fluid Management

Domagoj Mladinov, MD, PhD[a], Erin Isaza, BS[b], Andre F. Gosling, MD[c],
Adrienne L. Clark, MD[d], Jasleen Kukreja, MD, MPH[e], Marek Brzezinski, MD, PhD[f],*

KEYWORDS

- Fluid therapy • Resuscitation • Perioperative medicine • Anesthesia • Surgery
- Geriatrics

KEY POINTS

- Age-related decline in organ-specific reserves leads to increased hemodynamic instability and greater vulnerability to fluid shifts and electrolytes imbalances, making optimal perioperative fluid management of the aging patient challenging.
- There is limited generalizable evidence to guide perioperative fluid management in the geriatric patient, with robust clinical judgment remaining at the center of optimal fluid management.
- Perioperative fluid management strategies need to be restrictive and dynamically tailored to patient characteristics, severity of the surgical procedure, and blood loss.

INTRODUCTION

Perioperative fluid management has evolved over the last 25 years, starting with liberal fluid use in the early 2000s, followed by a restrictive approach in the second decade, to the current more balanced approach over the last 5 years.[1] The latter emerged as decrease in the volume of crystalloids administered was linked to an increase in acute kidney injury (AKI) incidence, particularly with resultant increase in vasopressor use.[1,2] Not surprisingly, given these swings in the *"pendulum"* of fluid management, the

[a] Department of Anesthesiology, Perioperative and Pain Medicine, Brigham and Women's Hospital, 75 Francis Street, CWN-L1, Boston, MA 02115, USA; [b] University of California, San Francisco, School of Medicine, 500 Parnassus Avenue, MU 405 W San Francisco, CA 94143, USA; [c] Department of Anesthesiology and Perioperative Medicine, University of Alabama at Birmingham, 619 19th Street South, JT 845D, Birmingham, AL 35249, USA; [d] Department of Anesthesia and Perioperative Care, University of California, 500 Parnassus Avenue, MU 405 W San Francisco, CA 94143, USA; [e] Division of Cardiothoracic Surgery, Department of Surgery, University of California, 500 Parnassus Avenue, MU 405 W San Francisco, CA 94143, USA; [f] Department of Anesthesia and Perioperative Care, University of California, VA Medical Center-San Francisco, 4150 Clement Street, San Francisco CA 94121, USA
* Corresponding author. VA Medical Center, Anesthesiology Service (129), 4150 Clement Street, San Francisco, CA 94121.
E-mail address: marek.brzezinski@ucsf.edu

Anesthesiology Clin 41 (2023) 613–629
https://doi.org/10.1016/j.anclin.2023.03.001
1932-2275/23/© 2023 Elsevier Inc. All rights reserved.

current clinical practices of perioperative fluid management, including volume status assessment, fluid choice, fluid administration strategies, or blood product use are characterized by a high degree of interindividual and interinstitutional controversy, heterogeneity, and bias.

Establishing optimal fluid management is particularly challenging in the elderly due to combination of age-related physiological changes in organ function, increased co-morbid burden, and larger fluid shifts frequently related to more complex surgical procedures.[3] Furthermore, many studies examining fluid management have focused on *critical care* patients and/or populations with a small to moderate geriatric cohort, thus limiting the generalizability of results for *perioperative* fluid management in the *geriatric* population.[4]

Thus, the goal of this manuscript was to review the available clinical evidence, followed by a concise, pragmatic, and critical appraisal of the data to answer several key questions relevant to everyday clinical practice when taking care of geriatric patients.

What Aspects to Consider in the Elderly?

A major factor of perioperative fluid management in the elderly is the age-related decline in organ function.[2–5] Especially, the reduction in cardiac and renal reserves may expose this cohort to higher risk of fluid and electrolytes imbalances or inadequate tissue perfusion leading to increased morbidity and mortality.[2–5]

Structural changes in the cardiovascular system associated with normal aging may include stiffening of the arteries, increasing left ventricular wall thickness and stiffening, diastolic dysfunction, degenerative changes of the heart valves, or the cardiac conduction system.[2–5] Furthermore, autonomic nervous system undergoes age-related changes ("dysautonomia of aging") that may include overactive sympathetic nervous system activity (SNA) impaired beta adrenoreceptor responsiveness, or decreased sensitivity of arterial baroreceptor reflex.[4–8] As a result, elderly patients may be at risk for increased hemodynamic instability and inadequate tissue perfusion:[3–5,9]

- *At induction:* Severe hypotension, due to combination of pronounced pharmacodynamic sensitivity to anesthetics, acute decrease in SNA, vasodilatation, and limited cardiac reserve, is common in this population, especially, in patients with mild preoperative hypovolemia which is characteristic for this cohort.
- *Intraoperatively:* Labile hemodynamics with increased dependence on preload and sinus rhythm (atrial kick) is common. Aging patients are at higher risk for ectopic beats, intraoperative arrhythmias, myocardial ischemia, disproportionally large variations in blood pressure from small-to-modest changes in cardiac filling, contractility, or electrolytes.
- *Postoperatively*: Removal of anesthetic agents, return of SNA to baseline, combined with intraoperative fluids, and postoperative surgical pain frequently result in hypertension. In addition, some may be at risk for pulmonary edema given the limited ability of the stiffened cardiovascular system to buffer any increase in intravascular volume.

Three key changes in the renal system associated with advancing age include progressive decrease in renal mass, renal blood flow, and total body renin and aldosterone levels.[2,4,5] Consequently, elderly patients demonstrate decreased ability to clear medications, handle excess fluid, or maintain appropriate intravascular volume.

In summary: The natural age-related decline in organ-specific reserves lead to increased hemodynamic instability, greater vulnerability to fluid shifts and electrolytes imbalances making optimal perioperative fluid management of the aging patient challenging.

How to Assess Intravascular Volume Status?

Monitoring of intravascular volume status is an essential step in ensuring appropriate fluid management. Most surgeries can be safely and successfully performed using the well-established noninvasive approach to fluid monitoring, including.

- Preinduction assessment in the awake patient: thirst, skin turgor, capillary refill time, urine output, lethargy, and postural dizziness.
- The use of standard continuous hemodynamic monitors, such as blood pressure, heart rate, and electrocardiogram (ECG)
- The continuous measurement of intraoperative fluid losses, including urine output, blood loss, and insensible fluid losses.

Complex surgical procedures, surgical patients with high comorbid burden, or unexpected perioperative challenges may require additional, more invasive methods to *monitor intravascular volume status* and predict fluid responsiveness.

- *Static hemodynamic* (eg, central venous pressure, pulmonary artery pressure, systemic arterial pressure, urine output) and *laboratory parameters* (eg, lactic acidosis, elevated serum lactate, or base deficit) provide only a suboptimal and unpredictable representation of the clinical volume status.[10–12] For example, oliguria is not always a sign of hypovolemia in the intraoperative setting, as it can represent a side effect of certain anesthetics or surgical stress itself.[13,14] The same applies to blood pressure and heart rate, given lack of a consistent correlation between blood pressure and cardiac output.[15] Similarly, the intermittent nature of intraoperative measurements of lactate and mixed-venous oxygen saturation make them poor markers of acute changes in volume status. Having said that, rising serum lactate and decreasing mixed-venous oxygen saturation are excellent markers of global tissue hypoperfusion and are frequently used when there is clinical uncertainty about the presence of ongoing global malperfusion as well as to help better define its clinical severity.
- *Dynamic hemodynamic parameters* have been found to consistently provide better assessment of volume responsiveness than traditional static parameters:[16–23]
  - The continuous assessment of *respiratory variations in arterial and/or venous pressure waveforms* has emerged as one of the most widely adopted approaches to intraoperative monitoring of fluid status, given its simplicity and reliability.[21,23–27] Commonly used examples include pulse pressure variation (PPV), stroke volume variation (SVV), systolic blood pressure variation (SBPV), and changes in the diameter of the inferior vena cava. During mechanical ventilation, increased intrathoracic pressure during inspiration leads to reduced venous return and consequently stroke volume. Assuming constant arterial vasomotor tone and cardiac function, pulse pressure, and systolic blood pressure will vary with the respiratory cycle.[27] Variation between inspiratory and expiratory measurements of greater than 10% to 15% was found to represent a reliable marker of intravascular volume depletion.[28,29] PPV and SBPV can generally be visually assessed or manually or automatically calculated. Visual assessment and calculation have been found to nearly always lead to similar treatment decisions.[21,24] Although superior to static hemodynamic parameters, PPV, and SVV reportedly have limited sensitivity and specificity,[30] suggesting that such dynamic indexes should be considered

in the clinical context when making treatment decisions.[21] Another limiting factor is that measurements of respiratory variations in pressure waveforms can be inaccurate when a patient is spontaneously breathing, when the tidal volume is less than 8 mL/kg, when the PEEP is high (>15 cm H_2O), and/or when the chest is open.[21,31–33]

- o *Ultrasound* is another option for dynamic monitoring of intravascular volume status, particularly when PPV and SBPV are inaccurate. Transesophageal Doppler ultrasound can be used to measure blood flow through the descending thoracic aorta,[23,34,35] whereas transesophageal and transthoracic echocardiography can be used to directly assess the intravascular volume status.[36,37]
- o Finally, there is a growing number of *technologies that measure cardiac output noninvasively* (eg, pleth variability index, thoracic electrical bioimpedance) or take advantage of an existing *indwelling arterial catheter* (pulse waveform analysis).[38–41] Although the ease and noninvasiveness of these devices makes them very attractive, their use remains limited due to high inaccuracy in measurement of cardiac output.[42]

In summary: Although a wide range of different approaches, techniques, and technologies have been introduced over the years, none has emerged as the uniformly accepted "gold standard." Thus, even in the year 2023, the best monitor of intravascular volume status in the elderly seems to be the experienced clinician, who by continuously integrating a wide range of tools, monitors, and observations in real-time, can obtain an accurate and dynamic representation of intraoperative fluid status.[4]

What Type of Fluid Should Be Used for Volume Resuscitation?

The optimal choice of type of intravenous fluid remains controversial. Multiple fluid therapies with sound theoretical rationale for their use are available. Yet, little evidence exists of their benefits in clinical practice. Hence, several have been used in clinical practice without a rigorous evaluation of outcomes.

In the last decade, the safety of 0.9% saline (commonly known as "normal saline") has been questioned, with some authors labeling it "abnormal saline."[43,44] Although the tonicity of 0.9% NaCl is similar to physiological levels, its chloride concentration far exceeds that of plasma, affecting the strong ion difference and driving metabolic acidosis.[45,46] In a study with healthy volunteers, renal cortical perfusion fell significantly from baseline after 0.9% NaCl infusion, but not after a balanced electrolyte solution.[47] Further, prospective trials have reported potential harm with 0.9% saline resuscitation compared with balanced crystalloids.[48,49] On the other hand, the saline versus plasma-lyte for ICU fluid Therapy (SPLIT) trial comparing effects of 0.9% saline and a balanced crystalloid solution in intensive care units (ICUs) on renal complications demonstrated similar rates of AKI or failure in the two groups.[50] Other notable studies addressing this question were SALT-ED, which assessed patients outside of the ICU, and SMART, which included critically ill patients.[49,51] Although saline against lactated ringers or plasma-lyte in the emergency department (SALT-ED) was a negative trial, balanced crystalloids versus saline in critically ill adults (SMART)reported a lower rate of composite outcome of death from any cause, new renal replacement therapy (RRT), or persistent renal dysfunction in the group that received balanced crystalloids. More recently, two large randomized trials (balanced solution versus saline in intensive care study [BaSICS] and plasma-lyte versus saline study [PLUS]) reported no differences in mortality between the two crystalloid solutions.[52,53] In a meta-analysis of randomized trials comprising over 35,000 patients, the investigators concluded that balanced crystalloids are most likely beneficial when compared with 0.9% NaCl, with an estimated effect that ranges from a 9% relative reduction to a 1% relative increase in the risk of death.[54]

In contrast to crystalloids, colloid solutions offer a theoretical advantage of requiring less volume to produce the same intravascular expansion. The saline versus albumin for fluid resuscitation in the critically ill (SAFE) trial evaluated albumin and saline as fluid therapies and demonstrated no difference in all-cause mortality at 28 days between the groups.[55] Similar results were noted in the volume replacement with albumin in severe sepsis (ALBIOS) trial in 28- and 90-day mortality.[56] Of note, the effects of albumin may differ depending on the subgroup of patient studied; in the SAFE trail, a nonsignificant trend of reduced mortality in the severe sepsis subgroup but a worse 28-day mortality in the traumatic brain injury (TBI) subgroup was observed with albumin, whereas a post hoc analysis of patients with septic shock in ALBIOS demonstrated a benefit only in 90-day mortality.[56–58] Additional studies found albumin to be harmful in patients with acute ischemic stroke, being associated with increased rates of intracerebral hemorrhage and pulmonary edema.[57]

With respect to synthetic colloids, high-quality randomized trials revealed the association of hydroxyethyl starch with an increased incidence of AKI, need for RRT, bleeding, and death.[58–62] Other synthetic formulations such as gelatins and dextrans have not been adequately tested for safety and they should be avoided due to concerns for adverse events.

In summary: (1) except for specific populations (such as patients with increased intracranial pressure, brain edema, or hyponatremia), the use of balanced crystalloids solutions is preferable; (2) current evidence does not support the use of albumin in critically ill patients and only suggest a potential benefit in patients with septic shock. Evidence advises against its administration in patients suffering from TBI or stroke; and (3) overall evidence advises against using synthetic colloids as volume expander therapy.

What Volume of Intravascular Fluids to Administer?

The expected blood loss, fluid shifts of the planned surgical procedure, and its complexity dictate the intraoperative fluid management strategy.

- In patients undergoing *brief minimally-to-moderately invasive surgery* who are expected to have rapid postoperative recovery (eg, outpatient or short floor stay), administration of 1 to 2 L of a balanced electrolyte solution over the course of the procedure has been found to decrease postoperative pain and nausea.[63,64] Naturally, this volume must be adjusted in patients at risk for volume overload.

- In patients undergoing *major invasive surgery*, there is inconsistent evidence as to what constitutes the best fluid management strategy, although there is a strong agreement on which strategies should not be recommended as they may *increase* the risk of perioperative complications:

  o Currently, recommended strategies, though the strength of evidence varies, include:

    ▪ *Restrictive (zero-balance) strategy for patients* with an expected blood loss of less than a liter: only fluids lost during surgery are replaced at approximately 3 mL/kg per hour with a balanced crystalloid (replacement of sensible and insensible losses) as well as additional fluid for blood loss.[11,12] Although many studies report superior outcomes with this approach,[11,12,65–68] there are some disconcerting data linking the restrictive fluid strategy with a higher risk of AKI,[69,70] highlighting the need for continuous intraoperative fluid monitoring to avoid hypovolemia.

- *Goal-directed therapy in patients undergoing major invasive surgery with expected significant blood loss:* In this approach, fluid is administered to reach a set-measured physiologic parameter, such as PPV/SBPV (estimated from intra-arterial waveform tracing), stroke volume (measured via esophageal Doppler), or left ventricle size (assessed via transesophageal echocardiography).[38] Similar to restrictive strategy, patients receive a continuous infusion of 3 mL/kg/h of a balanced crystalloid.[2,11] In addition, the patient's fluid responsiveness is assessed to maintain optimal intravascular volume status. This is typically accomplished using 250 to 500 mL boluses until the patient is no longer fluid responsive (ie, returned to the goal value of monitored physiologic parameter).[28,29] Although the data supporting goal-directed therapy have not been consistent,[71–77] the results of multiple meta-analyses suggest that the benefits of goal-directed therapy may be less in optimization of fluid responsiveness but more in optimizing tissue and organ perfusion.[78–80] Consistent with these results, a strategy that combined optimization of fluid responsiveness with optimization of cardiac output offered the biggest clinical benefit.[79,81,82]
- The *recommended ratios for blood loss replacement are 1.5:1 when using crystalloid and 1:1 when using colloid.*[2,55,83–87]
- *Vasopressors* should be considered to manage anesthesia-induced hypotension to avoid excess fluid administration.[88,89]
  - o Strategies that are currently NOT recommended, as they have been found to increase the risk of fluid overload and tissue and organ edema, ultimately leading to increased rates of adverse outcomes include:
    - Traditional liberal or pre-calculated fixed volume strategies, which typically account for preoperative deficits from fasting as well as intraoperative losses, including the nonanatomic "third space" loss.[11,12,90–96]
    - The administration of crystalloid in a 3:1 ratio to replace intraoperative blood loss.[83,87]
    - Excessively deep anesthesia (eg, bispectral index values < 40), increasing the risk of vasodilation and unnecessary fluid administration
    - Preloading with large volume of fluid before neuraxial blockade

In summary: Best perioperative fluid management strategies need to be restrictive and dynamically tailored to patient characteristics, the severity of the surgical procedure, and blood loss.[97–100]

When Is Blood Transfusion Indicated?

It is widely accepted that blood products are not to be considered as a volume expander therapy per se in non-hemorrhaging patients. The landmark TRICC trial demonstrated no mortality difference with a restrictive compared with liberal transfusion strategy in critically ill adult patients.[101] The trial was followed by multiple studies demonstrating non-inferior and in fact, some showing improved outcomes with a restrictive transfusion threshold of less than 7 to 8 g/dL.[102–104] However, optimal transfusion approaches in specific diseases and/or populations, such as elderly patients, have not been clearly established. Some data indicated increased risk of ischemia-related organ injury and mortality with restrictive transfusion, resulting in endorsement of a hemoglobin target of 9 g/dL in elderly patients undergoing hip fracture surgery.[105,106] Studies in oncologic patients showed mixed findings: some with survival trends favoring a higher hemoglobin threshold while others showing equal outcomes.[107,108]

With inconclusive or lacking evidence of optimizing transfusions of red blood cells based on hemoglobin levels, experts advocate basing the decision on the oxygen delivery/consumption balance.[109,110] Such approach would also take into consideration patient's characteristics (such as age, gender, and comorbidities) as well as underlying pathological processes. Studies describing cardiovascular and metabolic responses to isovolemic anemia offer a significant insight in assessing adequacy of oxygen delivery by using physiological and laboratory parameters such as stroke volume, heart rate, blood pressure, cardiac index, ECG changes, tissue oxygen saturation/cerebral oximetry, urine output, arterial and venous oxygen content, oxyhemoglobin saturation, and plasma lactate.[111,112] Two recent studies demonstrated that including mixed venous oxygen saturation into transfusion decision allowed for a more restrictive transfusion strategy without increasing the incidence of morbidity or mortality.[113,114] Another recent study examining the arterial-to-venous oxygen saturation (A-VO$_2$) difference as a surrogate for the oxygen delivery/consumption ratio indicated that transfusion in patients with higher A-VO$_2$ difference was associated with lower morbidity and mortality.[115]

In summary: A large proportion of hospitalized and critically ill patients receive transfusions. Guidelines that overall recommend restrictive red blood cell transfusion strategies are primarily based on hemoglobin concentration thresholds. However, in addition to hemoglobin concentration, decision to transfuse should be individualized and based on multiple other physiological and laboratory parameters with the ultimate goal of optimizing oxygen delivery.

When to Stop Fluid Resuscitation?

The goal of intravenous fluid therapy is to optimize intravascular volume and subsequently organ perfusion. The main indication for starting resuscitative fluid therapy is intravascular volume deficit or acute hypovolemia, though, duration of such therapy is frequently less clear.[116] Timely de-escalation of fluid therapy is of paramount importance to decrease the risk of fluid overload; excessive fluid can result in heart failure, worsening gas exchange, kidney function, and so forth and is associated with worse outcomes in critically ill patients.[117,118]

The decision on when to start and stop fluid therapy is not trivial in critically ill patients due to its dynamic nature, and some authors described it in four phases: resuscitation, optimization, stabilization, and de-escalation.[119]

- In the *resuscitation phase*, the focus is on lifesaving measures and correction of shock to obtain adequate organ perfusion. Early and rapid intravenous (IV) fluid administration is required in form of repeated boluses, which results in a *positive fluid balance*. A reasonable approach may entail administering a 3 to 4 mL/kg bolus over 10 to 15 min, repeated when necessary. The total amount of administered fluids is best individualized, rather than mandated by protocols.
- The second *optimization phase* is focused on organ rescue—optimization and maintenance of tissue perfusion and oxygenation. Fluid administration is more conservative, regularly reassessed with fluid challenge techniques, hemodynamic monitoring, and biochemical markers of perfusion. In this phase, a *neutral fluid balance* may be expected, with the goal of avoiding fluid overload.
- In the third *stabilization phase*, the focus is on organ support, with fluid therapy to ensure adequate water and electrolyte replacement. The aim is a *zero or negative fluid balance* with minimal maintenance infusion.

- Finally, the fourth *de-escalation phase* focuses on organ recovery. The main goal is mobilization of accumulated fluid, aiming for a *negative* fluid balance. If spontaneous diuresis is not adequate, active fluid removal with diuretics or ultrafiltration may be necessary.[119]

In summary: Fluid resuscitation is a dynamic process. Using a four-phase approach (resuscitation, optimization, stabilization, and de-escalation) emphasizes such dynamic nature of fluid resuscitation and particularly the importance of frequent reassessments and adjustments of therapies and therapeutic goals. It is recommended to reduce IV fluid therapy and consider stopping it during the optimization and stabilization phases, respectively.

Do Goal-Directed Fluid Management Strategies Make a Difference?

As discussed above, the aim of goal-directed fluid management is to improve organ perfusion and tissue oxygenation. Multiple factors can contribute to inadequate oxygen delivery (eg, reduced cardiac function, peripheral vascular resistance, or oxygen carrying capacity) and inadequate intravascular volume is only one of them. The relationship of intravascular volume contributing to the cardiac output is described by the Frank–Starling curve and may be considered the basis for goal-directed fluid resuscitation. Typically, fluid therapy is not the only therapy, but rather the first step in goal-directed approaches, which aims to achieve optimal volume status before adding inotropic or vasopressor therapy.

One of the first trials on the goal-directed therapy for treatment of severe sepsis and shock demonstrated decreased mortality with early goal-directed therapy.[120] However, besides fluid boluses, interventions included the use of vasopressors, dobutamine, and red blood cell transfusions, which makes it impossible to determine the impact of fluid therapies, regardless of other criticisms of that study. A randomized multicenter trial with patients who underwent major gastrointestinal surgery demonstrated that the use of cardiac output-guided hemodynamic therapy, which included IV fluids and inotropic medications, did not reduce complication or mortality rates.[72] This was in contrast to two trials: one in patients who underwent colorectal resection and another in low–moderate risk surgical patients that showed esophageal Doppler-guided goal-directed therapies were associated with reduced complications and hospital stay, with no mortality difference.[121,122] In these studies, the administration of fluids and vasoactive medications was guided by stroke volume, arterial blood pressure, and cardiac index. Interestingly, the studies found no difference in intraoperative or postoperative fluid or vasopressor administration. Therefore, the investigators speculated that the beneficial effects of esophageal Doppler-guided strategies were likely secondary to fluid administration at the right time.[121,122] A more recent trial showed that fluid management based on plethysmographic variability index in low-to-intermediate-risk orthopedic surgeries did not shorten hospitalization or improve complications.[41]

As the perioperative fluid therapy is considered one of the most important factors for postoperative outcomes, enhanced recovery after surgery (ERAS) protocols include multiple interventions that reduce the risk of intravascular fluid derangements. ERAS protocol-based studies failed to identify major benefits of goal-directed fluid therapy in abdominal surgery patients.[71] In addition to ERAS, another fluid management strategy—restricted fluid therapy—has been compared with goal-directed approaches. A meta-analysis of trials with patients who underwent noncardiac surgery concluded that it was uncertain whether restrictive fluid therapy is inferior to goal-directed fluid therapy.[123] The evidence was mainly based on studies including abdominal surgeries in a low-risk patient population.

In summary: Overall, variable benefits of goal-directed therapies have been reported, which may be attributed to heterogeneity between trials, study limitations, institutional differences in patient management, poorly defined endpoints, and difference in types of surgery. Evidence suggests that goal-directed fluid therapy may be beneficial only in certain populations; however, the treatment effect remains relatively small.[82] A recent systematic review and meta-analysis concluded that goal-directed hemodynamic therapy might reduce mortality and length of hospital stay with low certainty of evidence.[124] In regard to postoperative outcomes, only infection rate and anastomotic leakage reached moderate certainty of evidence.[124]

The "Third Space": Fact or Fiction?

The concept of the third space was proposed as a mechanism to explain reduction in extracellular fluid volume (ECV) commonly encountered during major surgical procedures or trauma that could not be accounted for by blood losses alone.[125,126] Third space losses have been further divided into anatomical and non-anatomical parts, though it is the non-anatomical extracellular space that is commonly considered as the "classic" third space. Given this separation from other spaces, third space has been described as a *"non-functional extra-cellular volume"*.[126,127]

The concept of the third space was originally popularized by a 1961 study, in which plasma volume, red blood cell mass, and ECVs were measured in a control group of patients undergoing minor procedures and an experimental group undergoing elective major surgical procedures.[125] The experimental group demonstrated a marked reduction in functional ECV compared with the control group. The investigators explained this loss through an internal redistribution of fluid into an area that no longer equilibrated with the extracellular fluid. Ultimately, these results led to widespread adoption of the concept of the third space with resultant liberal use of intraoperative fluid management.[128]

In recent years, the concept of third space as an actively consuming compartment has been increasingly challenged.[129] For one, there is a growing appreciation of increased morbidity risks associated with liberal approaches to perioperative fluid management, including respiratory complications, kidney injury, and electrolyte abnormalities.[93,96,130] Second, the methodology behind the studies originally describing the third space has been brought into question: A 2006 systematic review of tracer studies of ECV loss found that studies using longer equilibration times between the compartments failed to support the existence of the third space.[131]

The question about third space is further complicated by the fact that a recent body of literature demonstrated a fluid shift into a "space" not equilibrating with the plasma, that is, a compartment consistent with the definition of the third space. In fact, this line of research suggests that up to a third of the infused crystalloid fluid during surgery enters such a third space. The third space itself is proposed to represent a protective mechanism against intravascular fluid overload,[126] with potential sites including the gastrointestinal track, skin, surgical wounds, and lymphatics.[132] These losses have been shown to increase with isoflurane but not mechanical ventilation, possibly suggesting a link between inhalational anesthetics and perioperative fluid retention.[14]

In summary: The mystery of the elusive "third space" currently remains unsolved, although most of the evidence to date does not support its existence.

SUMMARY

Despite the growing importance, the evidence to guide perioperative fluid management in the elderly is still very limited. What has become clearer over the years, however, is that the best perioperative fluid management strategies need to be restrictive and dynamically tailored to patient characteristics, the severity of the surgical procedure, and blood loss.[97–100] A robust clinical judgment remains the fundamental core to optimal fluid management in this cohort in the perioperative period.

CLINICS CARE POINTS

- The natural age-related decline in organ-specific reserves lead to increased hemodynamic instability, greater vulnerability to fluid shifts and electrolytes imbalances.

- Although a wide range of different technologies has been introduced to monitor intravascular volume status, none has emerged as the uniformly accepted "gold standard", with the experienced clinician remaining as the best monitor of intravascular volume status in the elderly.

- Except for specific populations, the use of balanced crystalloids solutions is preferable. Current evidence does not support the use of albumin in critically ill patients and only suggest a potential benefit in patients with septic shock.

- Best perioperative fluid management strategies need to be restrictive and dynamically tailored to patient characteristics, the severity of the surgical procedure, and blood loss.

- Guidelines on red blood cell transfusion strategies are primarily based on hemoglobin concentration thresholds. However, in addition to hemoglobin concentration, decision to transfuse should be individualized and based on multiple other physiological and laboratory parameters with the ultimate goal of optimizing oxygen delivery.

- Goal-directed fluid therapy may be beneficial only in certain populations; however, the treatment effect remains relatively small.

- The four-phase approach to fluid resuscitation (resuscitation, optimization, stabilization and de-escalation) emphasizes the dynamic nature of fluid resuscitation and the necessity for frequent reassessments and adjustments of therapeutic goals.

REFERENCES

1. Chiu C, Fong N, Lazzareschi D, et al. Fluids, vasopressors, and acute kidney injury after major abdominal surgery between 2015 and 2019: a multicentre retrospective analysis. Br J Anaesth 2022;129:317–26.
2. Joshi G.P., UpToDate and O'Connor M.F., UpToDate, Waltham, MA.
3. Williams DGS, Aaron J, Koepke E, et al. Fluid Management in the Elderly. Current Anesthesiology Reports 2017;7:357–63.
4. Barnett S., UpToDate Joshi G.P., UpToDate, Waltham, MA.
5. Staheli B, Rondeau B. Anesthetic considerations in the geriatric population. Treasure island (FL): StatPearls; 2022.
6. Pfeifer MA, Weinberg CR, Cook D, et al. Differential changes of autonomic nervous system function with age in man. Am J Med 1983;75:249–58.
7. Ebert TJ, Morgan BJ, Barney JA, et al. Effects of aging on baroreflex regulation of sympathetic activity in humans. Am J Physiol 1992;263:H798–803.
8. Balasubramanian P, Hall D, Subramanian M. Sympathetic nervous system as a target for aging and obesity-related cardiovascular diseases. Geroscience 2019;41:13–24.
9. Brzezinski M, Rooke GA, Azocar RJ. Anesthetic Management. In: Rosenthal R, Zenilman M, Katlic M, editors. Principles and practice of geriatric surgery. Cham: Springer; 2017.

10. Joshi GP. Intraoperative fluid restriction improves outcome after major elective gastrointestinal surgery. Anesth Analg 2005;101:601–5.
11. Chappell D, Jacob M, Hofmann-Kiefer K, et al. A rational approach to perioperative fluid management. Anesthesiology 2008;109:723–40.
12. Brandstrup B. Fluid therapy for the surgical patient. Best Pract Res Clin Anaesthesiol 2006;20:265–83.
13. Brauer KI, Svensen C, Hahn RG, et al. Volume kinetic analysis of the distribution of 0.9% saline in conscious versus isoflurane-anesthetized sheep. Anesthesiology 2002;96:442–9.
14. Connolly CM, Kramer GC, Hahn RG, et al. Isoflurane but not mechanical ventilation promotes extravascular fluid accumulation during crystalloid volume loading. Anesthesiology 2003;98:670–81.
15. Kouz K, Bergholz A, Timmermann LM, et al. The Relation Between Mean Arterial Pressure and Cardiac Index in Major Abdominal Surgery Patients: A Prospective Observational Cohort Study. Anesth Analg 2022;134:322–9.
16. Ansari BM, Zochios V, Falter F, et al. Physiological controversies and methods used to determine fluid responsiveness: a qualitative systematic review. Anaesthesia 2016;71:94–105.
17. Cecconi M, Parsons AK, Rhodes A. What is a fluid challenge? Curr Opin Crit Care 2011;17:290–5.
18. Desebbe O, Cannesson M. Using ventilation-induced plethysmographic variations to optimize patient fluid status. Curr Opin Anaesthesiol 2008;21:772–8.
19. Funk DJ, Moretti EW, Gan TJ. Minimally invasive cardiac output monitoring in the perioperative setting. Anesth Analg 2009;108:887–97.
20. Magder S. Fluid status and fluid responsiveness. Curr Opin Crit Care 2010;16: 289–96.
21. Perel A. Using Dynamic Variables to Guide Perioperative Fluid Management. Anesthesiology 2020;133:929–35.
22. Renner J, Scholz J, Bein B. Monitoring fluid therapy. Best Pract Res Clin Anaesthesiol 2009;23:159–71.
23. Thiele RH, Bartels K, Gan TJ. Inter-device differences in monitoring for goal-directed fluid therapy. Can J Anaesth 2015;62:169–81.
24. Thiele RH, Colquhoun DA, Blum FE, et al. The ability of anesthesia providers to visually estimate systolic pressure variability using the "eyeball" technique. Anesth Analg 2012;115:176–81.
25. Si X, Xu H, Liu Z, et al. Does Respiratory Variation in Inferior Vena Cava Diameter Predict Fluid Responsiveness in Mechanically Ventilated Patients? A Systematic Review and Meta-analysis. Anesth Analg 2018;127:1157–64.
26. Monnet X, Marik PE, Teboul JL. Prediction of fluid responsiveness: an update. Ann Intensive Care 2016;6:111.
27. Jozwiak M, Monnet X, Teboul JL. Pressure Waveform Analysis. Anesth Analg 2018;126:1930–3.
28. Marik PE, Cavallazzi R, Vasu T, et al. Dynamic changes in arterial waveform derived variables and fluid responsiveness in mechanically ventilated patients: a systematic review of the literature. Crit Care Med 2009;37:2642–7.
29. Cannesson M, Le Manach Y, Hofer CK, et al. Assessing the diagnostic accuracy of pulse pressure variations for the prediction of fluid responsiveness: a "gray zone" approach. Anesthesiology 2011;115:231–41.
30. Messina A, Pelaia C, Bruni A, et al. Fluid Challenge During Anesthesia: A Systematic Review and Meta-analysis. Anesth Analg 2018;127:1353–64.

31. Raphael J, Regali LA, Thiele RH. Hemodynamic monitoring in thoracic surgical patients. Curr Opin Anaesthesiol 2017;30:7–16.
32. Michard F, Biais M. Rational fluid management: dissecting facts from fiction. Br J Anaesth 2012;108:369–71.
33. Jeong DM, Ahn HJ, Park HW, et al. Stroke Volume Variation and Pulse Pressure Variation Are Not Useful for Predicting Fluid Responsiveness in Thoracic Surgery. Anesth Analg 2017;125:1158–65.
34. Bisgaard J, Gilsaa T, Ronholm E, et al. Optimising stroke volume and oxygen delivery in abdominal aortic surgery: a randomised controlled trial. Acta Anaesthesiol Scand 2013;57:178–88.
35. Abbas SM, Hill AG. Systematic review of the literature for the use of oesophageal Doppler monitor for fluid replacement in major abdominal surgery. Anaesthesia 2008;63:44–51.
36. Reeves ST, Finley AC, Skubas NJ, et al, Council on Perioperative Echocardiography of the American Society of E, the Society of Cardiovascular A, Charleston SC, New York NY, Durham NC, Atlanta G and Boston M. Special article: basic perioperative transesophageal echocardiography examination: a consensus statement of the American Society of Echocardiography and the Society of Cardiovascular Anesthesiologists. Anesth Analg 2013;117:543–58.
37. Porter TR, Shillcutt SK, Adams MS, et al. Guidelines for the use of echocardiography as a monitor for therapeutic intervention in adults: a report from the American Society of Echocardiography. J Am Soc Echocardiogr 2015;28:40–56.
38. Zhang C. Does the Device Matter in Goal-Directed Fluid Therapy? Anesth Analg 2016;123:1061–2.
39. Saugel B, Thiele RH, Hapfelmeier A, et al. Technological Assessment and Objective Evaluation of Minimally Invasive and Noninvasive Cardiac Output Monitoring Systems. Anesthesiology 2020;133:921–8.
40. Kouz K, Scheeren TWL, de Backer D, et al. Pulse Wave Analysis to Estimate Cardiac Output. Anesthesiology 2021;134:119–26.
41. Fischer MO, Lemoine S, Tavernier B, et al. Hanouz JL and Optimization using the Pleth Variability Index Trial G. Individualized Fluid Management Using the Pleth Variability Index: A Randomized Clinical Trial. Anesthesiology 2020;133: 31–40.
42. Joosten A, Desebbe O, Suehiro K, et al. Accuracy and precision of non-invasive cardiac output monitoring devices in perioperative medicine: a systematic review and meta-analysisdagger. Br J Anaesth 2017;118:298–310.
43. Senussi MH. Abnormal saline: the unphysiological bag of brine. Crit Care 2014; 18:673.
44. Hayes W. Ab-normal saline in abnormal kidney function: risks and alternatives. Pediatr Nephrol 2019;34:1191–9.
45. Stewart PA. Modern quantitative acid-base chemistry. Can J Physiol Pharmacol 1983;61:1444–61.
46. Stewart PA. Independent and dependent variables of acid-base control. Respir Physiol 1978;33:9–26.
47. Chowdhury AH, Cox EF, Francis ST, et al. A randomized, controlled, double-blind crossover study on the effects of 2-L infusions of 0.9% saline and plasma-lyte(R) 148 on renal blood flow velocity and renal cortical tissue perfusion in healthy volunteers. Ann Surg 2012;256:18–24.
48. Yunos NM, Bellomo R, Hegarty C, et al. Association between a chloride-liberal vs chloride-restrictive intravenous fluid administration strategy and kidney injury in critically ill adults. JAMA 2012;308:1566–72.

49. Semler MW, Self WH, Wanderer JP, et al. Investigators S and the Pragmatic Critical Care Research G. Balanced Crystalloids versus Saline in Critically Ill Adults. N Engl J Med 2018;378:829–39.

50. Young P, Bailey M, Beasley R, et al. Effect of a Buffered Crystalloid Solution vs Saline on Acute Kidney Injury Among Patients in the Intensive Care Unit: The SPLIT Randomized Clinical Trial. JAMA 2015;314:1701–10.

51. Self WH, Semler MW, Wanderer JP, et al. Balanced Crystalloids versus Saline in Noncritically Ill Adults. N Engl J Med 2018;378:819–28.

52. Zampieri FG, Machado FR, Biondi RS, et al. Effect of Intravenous Fluid Treatment With a Balanced Solution vs 0.9% Saline Solution on Mortality in Critically Ill Patients: The BaSICS Randomized Clinical Trial. JAMA 2021;326:1–12.

53. Finfer S, Micallef S, Hammond N, et al. Investigators PS and the Australian New Zealand Intensive Care Society Clinical Trials G. Balanced Multielectrolyte Solution versus Saline in Critically Ill Adults. N Engl J Med 2022;386:815–26.

54. Hammond NE, Zampieri FG, Di Tanna GL, et al. Balanced Crystalloids versus Saline in Critically Ill Adults — A Systematic Review with Meta-Analysis, NEJM Evidence 2022;1:1–12.

55. Finfer S, Bellomo R, Boyce N, et al. A comparison of albumin and saline for fluid resuscitation in the intensive care unit. N Engl J Med 2004;350:2247–56.

56. Caironi P, Tognoni G, Masson S, et al. Albumin replacement in patients with severe sepsis or septic shock. N Engl J Med 2014;370:1412–21.

57. Martin RH, Yeatts SD, Hill MD, et al. Parts A and Investigators N. ALIAS (Albumin in Acute Ischemic Stroke) Trials: Analysis of the Combined Data From Parts 1 and 2. Stroke 2016;47:2355–9.

58. Brunkhorst FM, Engel C, Bloos F, et al. Intensive insulin therapy and pentastarch resuscitation in severe sepsis. N Engl J Med 2008;358:125–39.

59. Myburgh JA, Finfer S, Bellomo R, et al. Investigators C, Australian and New Zealand Intensive Care Society Clinical Trials G. Hydroxyethyl starch or saline for fluid resuscitation in intensive care. N Engl J Med 2012;367:1901–11.

60. Perner A, Haase N, Guttormsen AB, et al. Group ST and Scandinavian Critical Care Trials G. Hydroxyethyl starch 130/0.42 versus Ringer's acetate in severe sepsis. N Engl J Med 2012;367:124–34.

61. Rasmussen KC, Johansson PI, Hojskov M, et al. Hydroxyethyl starch reduces coagulation competence and increases blood loss during major surgery: results from a randomized controlled trial. Ann Surg 2014;259:249–54.

62. Schortgen F, Lacherade JC, Bruneel F, et al. Effects of hydroxyethylstarch and gelatin on renal function in severe sepsis: a multicentre randomised study. Lancet 2001;357:911–6.

63. Gan TJ, Belani KG, Bergese S, et al. Fourth Consensus Guidelines for the Management of Postoperative Nausea and Vomiting. Anesth Analg 2020;131:411–48.

64. Lambert KG, Wakim JH, Lambert NE. Preoperative fluid bolus and reduction of postoperative nausea and vomiting in patients undergoing laparoscopic gynecologic surgery. AANA J (Am Assoc Nurse Anesth) 2009;77:110–4.

65. Finfer S, Myburgh J, Bellomo R. Intravenous fluid therapy in critically ill adults. Nat Rev Nephrol 2018;14:541–57.

66. Lobo SM, Ronchi LS, Oliveira NE, et al. Restrictive strategy of intraoperative fluid maintenance during optimization of oxygen delivery decreases major complications after high-risk surgery. Crit Care 2011;15:R226.

67. Mahmooth Z, Jajja MR, Maxwell D, et al. Ultrarestrictive intraoperative intravenous fluids during pancreatoduodenectomy is not associated with an increase in post-operative acute kidney injury. Am J Surg 2020;220:264–9.

68. Rahbari NN, Zimmermann JB, Schmidt T, et al. Meta-analysis of standard, restrictive and supplemental fluid administration in colorectal surgery. Br J Surg 2009;96:331–41.

69. Furrer MA, Schneider MP, Loffel LM, et al. Impact of intra-operative fluid and noradrenaline administration on early postoperative renal function after cystectomy and urinary diversion: A retrospective observational cohort study. Eur J Anaesthesiol 2018;35:641–9.

70. Myles PS, Bellomo R, Corcoran T, et al. Australian, New Zealand College of Anaesthetists Clinical Trials N, the A and New Zealand Intensive Care Society Clinical Trials G. Restrictive versus Liberal Fluid Therapy for Major Abdominal Surgery. N Engl J Med 2018;378:2263–74.

71. Rollins KE, Lobo DN. Intraoperative Goal-directed Fluid Therapy in Elective Major Abdominal Surgery: A Meta-analysis of Randomized Controlled Trials. Ann Surg 2016;263:465–76.

72. Pearse RM, Harrison DA, MacDonald N, et al. Effect of a perioperative, cardiac output-guided hemodynamic therapy algorithm on outcomes following major gastrointestinal surgery: a randomized clinical trial and systematic review. JAMA 2014;311:2181–90.

73. Minto G, Scott MJ, Miller TE. Monitoring needs and goal-directed fluid therapy within an enhanced recovery program. Anesthesiol Clin 2015;33:35–49.

74. Miller TE, Roche AM, Mythen M. Fluid management and goal-directed therapy as an adjunct to Enhanced Recovery After Surgery (ERAS). Can J Anaesth 2015;62:158–68.

75. Joshi GP, Kehlet H. CON: Perioperative Goal-Directed Fluid Therapy Is an Essential Element of an Enhanced Recovery Protocol? Anesth Analg 2016; 122:1261–3.

76. Gomez-Izquierdo JC, Feldman LS, Carli F, et al. Meta-analysis of the effect of goal-directed therapy on bowel function after abdominal surgery. Br J Surg 2015;102:577–89.

77. Arslan-Carlon V, Tan KS, Dalbagni G, et al. Goal-directed versus Standard Fluid Therapy to Decrease Ileus after Open Radical Cystectomy: A Prospective Randomized Controlled Trial. Anesthesiology 2020;133:293–303.

78. Joosten A, Rinehart J, Van der Linden P, et al. Computer-assisted Individualized Hemodynamic Management Reduces Intraoperative Hypotension in Intermediate- and High-risk Surgery: A Randomized Controlled Trial. Anesthesiology 2021;135:258–72.

79. Deng QW, Tan WC, Zhao BC, et al. Is goal-directed fluid therapy based on dynamic variables alone sufficient to improve clinical outcomes among patients undergoing surgery? A meta-analysis. Crit Care 2018;22:298.

80. Chong MA, Wang Y, Berbenetz NM, et al. Does goal-directed haemodynamic and fluid therapy improve peri-operative outcomes?: A systematic review and meta-analysis. Eur J Anaesthesiol 2018;35:469–83.

81. Kaufmann T, Saugel B, Scheeren TWL. Perioperative goal-directed therapy - What is the evidence? Best Pract Res Clin Anaesthesiol 2019;33:179–87.

82. Maheshwari K, Sessler DI. Goal-directed Therapy: Why Benefit Remains Uncertain. Anesthesiology 2020;133:5–7.

83. Hartog CS, Kohl M, Reinhart K. A systematic review of third-generation hydrox-yethyl starch (HES 130/0.4) in resuscitation: safety not adequately addressed. Anesth Analg 2011;112:635–45.

84. He H, Liu D, Ince C. Colloids and the Microcirculation. Anesth Analg 2018;126: 1747–54.

85. McLean DJ, Shaw AD. Intravenous fluids: effects on renal outcomes. Br J Anaesth 2018;120:397–402.

86. Orbegozo Cortes D, Gamarano Barros T, Njimi H, et al. Crystalloids versus col-loids: exploring differences in fluid requirements by systematic review and meta-regression. Anesth Analg 2015;120:389–402.

87. Yates DR, Davies SJ, Milner HE, et al. Crystalloid or colloid for goal-directed fluid therapy in colorectal surgery. Br J Anaesth 2014;112:281–9.

88. Bellomo R. Noradrenaline: friend or foe? Heart Lung Circ 2003;12(Suppl 2): S42–8.

89. Sear JW. Kidney dysfunction in the postoperative period. Br J Anaesth 2005;95: 20–32.

90. Bundgaard-Nielsen M, Holte K, Secher NH, et al. Monitoring of peri-operative fluid administration by individualized goal-directed therapy. Acta Anaesthesiol Scand 2007;51:331–40.

91. Bundgaard-Nielsen M, Secher NH, Kehlet H. Liberal' vs. 'restrictive' periopera-tive fluid therapy–a critical assessment of the evidence. Acta Anaesthesiol Scand 2009;53:843–51.

92. Hamilton MA, Cecconi M, Rhodes A. A systematic review and meta-analysis on the use of preemptive hemodynamic intervention to improve postoperative out-comes in moderate and high-risk surgical patients. Anesth Analg 2011;112: 1392–402.

93. Hatton GE, Du RE, Wei S, et al. Positive Fluid Balance and Association with Post-Traumatic Acute Kidney Injury. J Am Coll Surg 2020;230:190–199 e1.

94. Lassen K. Intravenous fluid therapy. Br J Surg 2009;96:123–4.

95. Lobo DN. Fluid overload and surgical outcome: another piece in the jigsaw. Ann Surg 2009;249:186–8.

96. Shin CH, Long DR, McLean D, et al. Effects of Intraoperative Fluid Management on Postoperative Outcomes: A Hospital Registry Study. Ann Surg 2018;267: 1084–92.

97. Myles PS, Andrews S, Nicholson J, et al. Contemporary Approaches to Periop-erative IV Fluid Therapy. World J Surg 2017;41:2457–63.

98. Som A, Maitra S, Bhattacharjee S, et al. Goal directed fluid therapy decreases postoperative morbidity but not mortality in major non-cardiac surgery: a meta-analysis and trial sequential analysis of randomized controlled trials. J Anesth 2017;31:66–81.

99. Weinberg L, Mackley L, Ho A, et al. Impact of a goal directed fluid therapy al-gorithm on postoperative morbidity in patients undergoing open right hepatec-tomy: a single centre retrospective observational study. BMC Anesthesiol 2019; 19:135.

100. Zorrilla-Vaca A, Mena GE, Ripolles-Melchor J, et al. Goal-Directed Fluid Therapy and Postoperative Outcomes in an Enhanced Recovery Program for Colorectal Surgery: A Propensity Score-Matched Multicenter Study. Am Surg 2021;87: 1189–95.

101. Hebert PC, Wells G, Blajchman MA, et al. A multicenter, randomized, controlled clinical trial of transfusion requirements in critical care. Transfusion

Requirements in Critical Care Investigators, Canadian Critical Care Trials Group. N Engl J Med 1999;340:409–17.

102. Walsh TS, Boyd JA, Watson D, et al. Restrictive versus liberal transfusion strategies for older mechanically ventilated critically ill patients: a randomized pilot trial. Crit Care Med 2013;41:2354–63.

103. Mazer CD, Whitlock RP, Fergusson DA, et al. Investigators T and Perioperative Anesthesia Clinical Trials G. Restrictive or Liberal Red-Cell Transfusion for Cardiac Surgery. N Engl J Med 2017;377:2133–44.

104. Holst LB, Haase N, Wetterslev J, et al. Group TT and Scandinavian Critical Care Trials G. Lower versus higher hemoglobin threshold for transfusion in septic shock. N Engl J Med 2014;371:1381–91.

105. Hovaguimian F, Myles PS. Restrictive versus Liberal Transfusion Strategy in the Perioperative and Acute Care Settings: A Context-specific Systematic Review and Meta-analysis of Randomized Controlled Trials. Anesthesiology 2016;125: 46–61.

106. Griffiths R, Babu S, Dixon P, et al. Guideline for the management of hip fractures 2020: Guideline by the Association of Anaesthetists. Anaesthesia 2021;76: 225–37.

107. Tay J, Allan DS, Chatelain E, et al. Liberal Versus Restrictive Red Blood Cell Transfusion Thresholds in Hematopoietic Cell Transplantation: A Randomized, Open Label, Phase III, Noninferiority Trial. J Clin Oncol 2020;38:1463–73.

108. Bergamin FS, Almeida JP, Landoni G, et al. Liberal Versus Restrictive Transfusion Strategy in Critically Ill Oncologic Patients: The Transfusion Requirements in Critically Ill Oncologic Patients Randomized Controlled Trial. Crit Care Med 2017;45:766–73.

109. Spitalnik SL, Triulzi D, Devine DV, et al. Glynn S and State of the Science in Transfusion Medicine Working G. 2015 proceedings of the National Heart, Lung, and Blood Institute's State of the Science in Transfusion Medicine symposium. Transfusion 2015;55:2282–90.

110. Levy JH, Steiner ME. How to interpret recent restrictive transfusion trials in cardiac surgery: More new data or new more data? J Thorac Cardiovasc Surg 2019;157:1038–40.

111. Weiskopf RB, Viele MK, Feiner J, et al. Human cardiovascular and metabolic response to acute, severe isovolemic anemia. JAMA 1998;279:217–21.

112. Leung JM, Weiskopf RB, Feiner J, et al. Electrocardiographic ST-segment changes during acute, severe isovolemic hemodilution in humans. Anesthesiology 2000;93:1004–10.

113. Zeroual N, Blin C, Saour M, et al. Restrictive Transfusion Strategy after Cardiac Surgery. Anesthesiology 2021;134:370–80.

114. Fischer MO, Guinot PG, Debroczi S, et al. Individualised or liberal red blood cell transfusion after cardiac surgery: a randomised controlled trial. Br J Anaesth 2022;128:37–44.

115. Fogagnolo A, Taccone FS, Vincent JL, et al. Using arterial-venous oxygen difference to guide red blood cell transfusion strategy. Crit Care 2020;24:160.

116. Malbrain M, Langer T, Annane D, et al. Intravenous fluid therapy in the perioperative and critical care setting: Executive summary of the International Fluid Academy (IFA). Ann Intensive Care 2020;10:64.

117. Silva JM Jr, de Oliveira AM, Nogueira FA, et al. The effect of excess fluid balance on the mortality rate of surgical patients: a multicenter prospective study. Crit Care 2013;17:R288.

118. Acheampong A, Vincent JL. A positive fluid balance is an independent prognostic factor in patients with sepsis. Crit Care 2015;19:251.
119. Hoste EA, Maitland K, Brudney CS, et al. Four phases of intravenous fluid therapy: a conceptual model. Br J Anaesth 2014;113:740–7.
120. Rivers E, Nguyen B, Havstad S, et al. Tomlanovich M and Early Goal-Directed Therapy Collaborative G. Early goal-directed therapy in the treatment of severe sepsis and septic shock. N Engl J Med 2001;345:1368–77.
121. Noblett SE, Snowden CP, Shenton BK, et al. Randomized clinical trial assessing the effect of Doppler-optimized fluid management on outcome after elective colorectal resection. Br J Surg 2006;93:1069–76.
122. Calvo-Vecino JM, Ripolles-Melchor J, Mythen MG, et al. Effect of goal-directed haemodynamic therapy on postoperative complications in low-moderate risk surgical patients: a multicentre randomised controlled trial (FEDORA trial). Br J Anaesth 2018;120:734–44.
123. Wrzosek A, Jakowicka-Wordliczek J, Zajaczkowska R, et al. Perioperative restrictive versus goal-directed fluid therapy for adults undergoing major non-cardiac surgery. Cochrane Database Syst Rev 2019;12:CD012767.
124. Jessen MK, Vallentin MF, Holmberg MJ, et al. Goal-directed haemodynamic therapy during general anaesthesia for noncardiac surgery: a systematic review and meta-analysis. Br J Anaesth 2022;128:416–33.
125. Shires T, Williams J, Brown F. Acute change in extracellular fluids associated with major surgical procedures. Ann Surg 1961;154:803–10.
126. Hahn RG. Fluid escapes to the "third space" during anesthesia, a commentary. Acta Anaesthesiol Scand 2020;65(4):451–6.
127. Strunden MS, Heckel K, Goetz AE, et al. Perioperative fluid and volume management: physiological basis, tools and strategies. Ann Intensive Care 2011; 1:2.
128. Frost EA. The rise and fall of the third space: appropriate intraoperative fluid management. J Med Assoc Thai 2013;96:1001–8.
129. Jacob M, Chappell D, Rehm M. The 'third space'–fact or fiction? Best Pract Res Clin Anaesthesiol 2009;23:145–57.
130. Wang TJ, Pai KC, Huang CT, et al. A Positive Fluid Balance in the First Week Was Associated With Increased Long-Term Mortality in Critically Ill Patients: A Retrospective Cohort Study. Front Med 2022;9:727103.
131. Brandstrup B, Svensen C, Engquist A. Hemorrhage and operation cause a contraction of the extracellular space needing replacement–evidence and implications? A systematic review. Surgery 2006;139:419–32.
132. Hahn RG. Understanding volume kinetics. Acta Anaesthesiol Scand 2020;64: 570–8.

Data Science and Geriatric Anesthesia Research
Opportunity and Challenges

Mani Ratnesh S. Sandhu, MD[a,1], Mayanka Tickoo, MD, MS[b],
Amit Bardia, MBBS, MPH[c],*

KEYWORDS

- Clinical outcome • Geriatric anesthesia • Geriatric perioperative • Machine learning
- Deep learning • Data

KEY POINTS

- There is a tremendous need for research focusing on geriatric perioperative medicine.
- Big data research helps address the knowledge deficit by providing valuable information to guide clinical geriatric care and clinical trials.
- Wearable devices, machine and deep learning tools, visual analytics are novel sophisticated methodologies, which can be used in geriatric perioperative research.
- Low recruitment and retention rates, maintaining data security, and privacy are the key challenges faced by geriatric data scientists.

INTRODUCTION

Advancement in medicine during the past few decades has significantly increased the average life span of Americans. Based on recent census, the number of adults aged 65 years and older is about 46 million, and by 2060, this population is projected to double.[1] These trends carry major implications in anesthesiology. There is a steady increase in the number of patients in the geriatric cohort undergoing anesthesia for major and minor procedures. A recent web-based survey conducted among 1737 US-based physician anesthesiologist demonstrated that nearly all respondents provide anesthesia to adults aged 65 years and older, with a majority indicating that geriatric patients constituted 50% or more of their cases.[1,2] In fact, 35% of all inpatient

[a] Department of Neurosurgery, University of Iowa Hospitals and Clinics, Iowa City, IA, USA;
[b] Division of Pulmonary, Department of Medicine, Critical Care and Sleep Medicine, Tufts Medical Center, Biewend Building, 3Road Floor, 260 Tremont Street, Boston, MA 02118, USA;
[c] Department of Anesthesiology, Critical Care and Pain Medicine, Massachusetts General Hospital, Boston, MA 06520, USA
[1] Present address: 345 Clark Dr, Coralville, Iowa City, Iowa 52241, USA.
* Corresponding author. White 5, 55 Fruit street, Boston, MA 02114.
E-mail address: abardia@partners.org

Anesthesiology Clin 41 (2023) 631–646
https://doi.org/10.1016/j.anclin.2023.03.002
1932-2275/23/© 2023 Elsevier Inc. All rights reserved.
anesthesiology.theclinics.com

and 32% of all outpatient surgeries performed in the United States comprise of geriatric patients.[2] Therefore, ensuring high-quality and evidence-based care to older adults is a vital component of clinical care by anesthesiologists.[3]

Older adults are at a higher risk for perioperative complications with risks that largely correlate with an increase in age. Apart from major cardiovascular and pulmonary complications, surgeries on geriatric adults are associated with postoperative delirium, cognitive disorders, decline in functional status and increase in frailty, health-care utilization, and mortality.[4,5] Major medical organizations across the globe have recognized the distinct needs of the geriatric population and are promoting benchmarking initiatives to provide specific recommendations for perioperative care of older adults. However, owing to a lack of research specifically focused on geriatric patients, there is a paucity of high-quality evidence to support guidelines.

Advances in electronic health records have significantly increased the availability of high-quality information and reliable data. Driven by mandates including Health Information Technology for Economic and Clinical Health Act, we now have access to numerous databases focusing on diverse populations. Major perioperative efforts in the United States include, but are not limited to, the National Surgical Quality Program (NSQIP), the Society of Thoracic Surgeons National Database, the Closed Claims Registry of settled malpractice cases, the Multicenter Perioperative Outcomes Group (MPOG), the Anesthesia Quality Institute (AQI)'s National Anesthesia Clinical Outcomes Registry (NACOR), and Premier Healthcare databases (PHDs). Analyses of these robust national and private databases can provide multiparametric geriatric patient data, which can be used to generate evidence for health-care policies, creating risk stratification tools and modeling for future prospective studies.

In this article, we review available databases that can be used to perform meaningful research in geriatric anesthesia. We also highlight scientific topics related to geriatric anesthesiology and perioperative care and how readily available information can be exploited to provide results that promote accurate and reliable clinical decision-making.

WHAT IS DATA SCIENCE?

Data science is an interdisciplinary field that uses scientific algorithms, processes, and systems to extrapolate knowledge from structured or unstructured data. This field uses statistical, data management, and visualization skills to produce practical information from unorganized and organized data efficiently. This umbrella term includes various techniques used when extracting data and information. Health-care data can comprise information from government agencies, patient portals, Elctronic Health Records (EHR), wearable devices, research studies, and payer records. Below, we discuss some of the datasets that are commonly used in perioperative research and can be further exploited to specifically advance geriatric perioperative research (**Table 1**).

TYPES OF DATABASES
Administrative Datasets

In the process of providing and paying for health care, organizations generate administrative data on the population's characteristics and the type of services provided. Therefore, every encounter in health care contributes to administrative data. The information is collected from various sources, such as insurance claims and providers' systems.[6] Although the primary purpose of these datasets is operational in nature, the vast clinical information thus accumulated has been exploited to generate

Table 1
Commonly utilized databases that can be used for perioperative research in geriatric patients

Database	Description	URL
Administrative or claims data		
Anesthesia Close Claims Project (CCP)	CCP project to closely analyze malpractice claims and trends in anesthesia-related patient safety topics	https://www.aqihq.org/accmain.aspx
Comparative Benchmarking System database (CRICO)	CRICO includes of all Harvard medical institutions and their affiliates covering 35 hospitals providing data in an effort decrease medical errors and malpractice claims	https://www.rmf.harvard.edu/About-CRICO
HCUP	HCUP is the most comprehensive source of hospital care data providing inpatient stays, ambulatory surgery, service visits and emergency department visits	https://www.ahrq.gov/data/hcup/index.html
Manufacturer and User Facility Device Experience (MAUDE) database	MAUDE database houses medical device reports submitted to FDA by mandatory reporter	https://www.accessdata.fda.gov/scripts/cdrh/cfdocs/cfmaude/search.cfm
Medicaid	Medicaid databases provide data on drug pricing and payment, enrollment, quality, and state drug utilization	https://data.medicaid.gov
Medicare or Medical Coverage Database	Medical Coverage Database contains national and local coverage documents	https://data.cms.gov
Ontario administrative data	This database consists of multiple record-level and linkable health datasets providing information on drug claims, hospital and emergency stay, and claims for home and long-term care	https://www.ices.on.ca/Data-and-Privacy/ICES-data
Optum	Optum is an American pharmacy benefit manager maintained by UnitedHealth Group providing information on drug claims	https://www.optum.com/business/life-sciences/real-world-data/claims-data.html
Premier	PHD is private US hospital-based, service-level, all-payer database that contains information mainly on in-patient discharge	https://products.premierinc.com/downloads/PremierHealthcareDatabaseWhitepaper.pdf

(continued on next page)

Table 1
(continued)

Database	Description	URL
The Marketscan Databases	The MarketScan databases contain data on inpatient and outpatient claims, outpatient prescription claims, clinical utilization records, and health-care expenditures	https://marketscan.truvenhealth.com/marketscanportal/
Clinical Registries		
MPOG	MPOG database provides information on about 20 million cases, 327 million medication records, and 43 billion physiologic observations	https://mpog.org
NACOR	Apart from collecting demographics, diagnostic and procedural coding, and provider information, NACOR also collects detailed information on anesthesia procedures	https://www.aqihq.org/introduction-to-nacor.aspx
National Cardiovascular Data Registry (NCDR)	Limited datasets from NCDR are available for cardiovascular research to identify risk factors and outcomes, procedure, and treatment trends	https://cvquality.acc.org/NCDR-Home
National Surgical Quality Improvement Program (ACS-NSIQP)	Large comprehensive risk-adjusted surgical data from patient's medical charts	https://www.facs.org/quality-programs/data-and-registries/acs-nsqip/
National Trauma Data Bank (NTDB)	NTDB is the largest aggregation of US trauma registry data ever assembled providing information on outcomes of trauma patients	https://www.facs.org/quality-programs/trauma/quality/national-trauma-data-bank/
National Health and Nutrition Examination Survey (NHANES)	This program uniquely combines interviews and physical examination to assess health and nutritional status of children and adults	https://www.cdc.gov/nchs/nhanes/index.htm
Miscellaneous		
Multiparameter Intelligent Monitoring in Intensive Care II (MIMIC - II)	This database consists of 25,328 intensive care unit status including granular details such vital signs trends and waveforms, drip rates, and ventilator settings	https://www.ncbi.nlm.nih.gov/pmc/articles/PMC3124312/

Data from Zhong, H., et al., An Overview of Commonly Used Data Sources in Observational Research in Anesthesia. Anesth Analg, 2022. 134(3): p. 548-558.

meaningful clinical evidence. We focus here on a few datasets, which have enabled research on a broad range of health policies, access, cost, and quality of different health services, and outcomes of treatments at individual, hospital, state, and national levels.

Healthcare Cost and Utilization Project (HCUP) consists of several health-care databases and related analytical tools developed through a collaboration between federal and state health-care industry and is sponsored by the Agency for Healthcare Research and Quality.[7] HCUP includes the largest collection of all payer encounter level data bought together by state and federal data organizations, hospital associations, and private data organizations beginning in 1988. HCUP databases include National Inpatient Sample (NIS), the largest publicly available all-payer inpatient database in the United States, with information on almost 7 million hospital stays each year. With surgical inpatient data representing a significant chunk of inpatient discharges from community hospitals, NIS has been commonly used to identify and track trends in perioperative care.[8] Other datasets included in HCUP are the Nationwide Ambulatory Surgery Sample,[9] Nationwide Readmissions Database, State Inpatient Databases, and State Ambulatory Surgery and Services Databases. Given the diversity and large sample size of HCUP datasets, studies have addressed a broad range of perioperative questions. For example, association of insurance type on outcomes after inpatient shoulder arthroplasty,[10] cardiovascular outcomes among older adults,[11] and incidence and risk factors associated with local anesthetic systemic toxicity in total joint arthroplasty[12] while being less affected by selection bias.[8]

PHD is a private US hospital-based, service-level, all-payer database that contains information on inpatient discharges, primarily from nonprofit, nongovernmental and community and teaching hospitals catering to both urban and rural populations.[13] The PHD contains data covering 121 million inpatient visits and 897 million outpatient encounters from approximately 231 million unique patients.[13] Although PHD is not nationally representative because it only includes about 1000 hospitals, the granular data provided by this database is ideal for pharmaco-epidemiological studies.[14] Data comprise demographics, detailed charges per patient, current procedural terminology and international classification of diseases (ICD) diagnosis and procedural codes, standard readmission data, and general laboratory and microbiology data for select hospital encounters. The detailed coding and charges data in this database has been used to conduct studies to investigate the impact of use of different analgesics in colectomies,[15] hip and knee arthroplasties,[16] and spine surgeries[17] to describe variations in use of perioperative multimodal analgesic therapies and describe the incidence of postoperative delirium in patients undergoing lower extremity joint arthroplasty.[18]

Other administrative databases include the state-level Ontario Healthcare Administrative Databases (including data on insurance plan claims, drug benefits claims, ambulatory care, and discharges). This is one of the most widely used datasets in perioperative research.[6,14] Some other private databases include data from Optum, a subsidiary of UnitedHealth Group, focusing on pharmacy and health-care solutions, and The MarketScan Databases that include databases from patients with employer-based health insurance, Medicare beneficiaries who possess supplemental insurance from their employers and patients with Medicaid in select states.[19] A few studies originating from these datasets include the association of polypharmacy with clinical outcomes after elective noncardiac surgery,[20] the association of frailty in the geriatric population after elective surgery,[21] the role of opioid use in promoting perioperative psychiatric comorbidities,[22] and the impact of perioperative epidural placement in patients undergoing abdominal surgery.[23]

Clinical Registries

Clinical registries are databases that systematically collect health-care information focusing on specific diseases or procedures and related clinical outcomes. In contrast to administrative data, clinical registries can provide more relevant clinical information and a more comprehensive range of information on comorbidities and outcomes.[24] However, participation in these registries is usually voluntary and involves costly resources for data entry, which may introduce biases in observational studies conducted using these databases. Nonetheless, many such registries have been used to advance perioperative research.

The American College of Surgeons (ACS) NSQIP is a nationwide outcomes-based program involving about 700 hospitals primarily intended to measure and improve the quality of surgical care. It uses a prospective database to quantify 30-day, risk and case-mix adjusted outcomes, and records variables pertinent to surgical care such as demographics, anesthetic type, comorbidities, and postoperative complications. NSQIP data have found extensive use in perioperative research, including studies comparing attributable mortality of postoperative bleeding with mortality associated with postoperative venous thromboembolism,[25] anesthetic type and clinical outcomes of patients undergoing traumatic fractures,[26] and development of risk scores to predict delirium in patients with hip fracture.[27]

In 2008, the American Society of Anesthesiologists (ASA) chartered the AQI to develop the NACOR.[28] NACOR accepts case-level administrative and clinical data from voluntary participating anesthesia practices including health maintenance organizations and the Department of Defense or Veteran Affairs. Apart from collecting demographics, diagnostic and procedural coding, and provider information, NACOR also collects detailed information on anesthesia procedures thus, providing a unique dataset to study specific anesthetic techniques and their trends across different systems. Some of the studies from this dataset include usage of peripheral nerve block in mastectomy and lumpectomy,[29] patterns of utilization of interscalene nerve blocks for total shoulder arthroplasty,[30] and variability in case durations for certain common surgical procedures.[31]

Another unique source of data in perioperative research is the MPOG. This nonprofit academic consortium was started by the University of Michigan in 2008 and has now greatly expanded to include 51 hospitals across 21 states and 2 countries and has more than 13.6 million anesthetic cases. MPOG database provides granular intraoperative data, which includes more than 5 billion vital signs and 125 million laboratory values.[32] Some of the studies originating from this dataset include the role of intubation rescue techniques after failed direct laryngoscopy,[33] role of alarm limits for intraoperative drug infusions,[34] and investigating low tidal volume regimen in lung resection surgery.[35]

Translational Data and Biobanks

Geriatric anesthesia is characterized by highly complex patients, for whom personalization of treatment can be beneficial. Recent advances and adoption of robust data infrastructures aimed at aggregating and bridging multiparametric patient data have supported the emergence of personalized medicine. One of the pillars for such practice is biobanks—rapidly pooling reliable biological samples, which can be available for pathophysiological description, and identifying biomarkers for treatment effectiveness and outcomes.[36] The Anesthetic Biobank of Cerebrospinal fluid is a unique repository aiming to investigate cerebrospinal fluid (CSF)-based candidate biomarkers and neuropsychiatric symptoms.[37] Although not for geriatric population, the Uniformed Services

University Pain Registry Biobank is an exciting platform linking patient-reported outcomes to molecular mechanisms underlying acute and chronic pain.[38] Perhaps, a similar repository can be developed in collaboration with the Department of Defense and Veteran affairs to focus on older adults.

OPPORTUNITIES IN GERIATRIC ANESTHESIA RESEARCH
Frailty and Risk Stratification

Frailty has been conceptually defined as a state of increased vulnerability, a syndrome of decreased physiologic reserve and resistance to stressors.[39] Frailty in surgical patients can lead to increased adverse outcomes, such as loss of mobility and independence.[40] Frailty is especially relevant in older adults with an incidence of 9% in 75 to 79-year-olds and 26% for those aged older than 85 years.[41] Frail older individuals are vulnerable to geriatric syndromes including functional decline, mobility impairment, polypharmacy, delirium, dementia, pressure ulcers, falls, malnutrition and incontinence, all of which have an impact on postoperative recovery. Therefore, optimal perioperative care should include the identification of frailty, a multisystem and multidisciplinary evaluation preoperatively, and discussion of treatment goals and expectations.

Although the importance of recognizing frailty in perioperative care, there is no consensus on how it should be measured. To date, clinicians rely on instinct and experience to identify frail patients. This "eyeballing" technique can be subjective with large interobserver variability.[42] Some of commonly used, however, not universally adopted frailty indices are mentioned here. One example is the modified Frailty Index (mFI), which includes history of diabetes, hypertension, congestive heart failure (CHF), chronic obstructive pulmonary disease (COPD), and dependent functional status.[43] The Charlson Comorbidity Index is another example of frailty scoring system, which unlike mFI, weighs certain comorbidities based on their prognostic values.[44] The "phenotype" model also known as the Cardiovascular Health Study relies on changes in lean body mass, strength, endurance, walking performance, and activity level[39] is another commonly used method to classify a patient frail.

The American Geriatric Society recommends that the preoperative assessment of older patients include a multisystem, multidisciplinary evaluation, which extends beyond the standard preoperative assessment to include treatment goals and expectations.[45] Using institutional and national level data, risk stratification tools can be developed to optimize preoperative assessments in older adults.

Clinical Outcomes

Outcomes are the endpoints that are monitored during a study to demonstrate the impact of an intervention or exposure in a select population. Clinical outcomes commonly include hospital complications, length of stay, discharge disposition, the total cost per admission, in-hospital mortality, and readmission. With the increasing availability of data sources, many observational studies have emerged showing the association of age with adverse outcomes, including after cardiac and noncardiac surgery.[4,21,46–51] Studies have shown significantly higher odds of developing postoperative pulmonary[52] and cardiac complications,[53,54] acute kidney disease[55] and mortality in an older population, with risk increasing with age.[48,52] Advanced age is also associated with the development of postoperative delirium, with the highest incidence after emergency, cardiac, or orthopedic surgeries.[56,57] Notably, 40% of these patients never return to their neurocognitive baseline.[57,58] The ICD-10 manuals now have codes explicitly related to anesthesia and anesthetics, thereby allowing the identification of anesthesia-related morbidity and mortality. A study on about 106 million patients undergoing surgery demonstrated that anesthesia-related issues caused death in 8 per million surgical patients, with the advanced age group exhibiting the highest death rate.[58]

Although advanced age seems to be a common risk factor for adverse outcomes and mortality after a procedure, it is by no means the sole predictor of adverse events. The presence of different comorbidities as well as types and length of procedure are well-established predictors[4,46] of adverse outcomes. In fact, older age has not definitively proven to independently increase the risk of postoperative cardiac-related complications or mortality and is considered a minor risk factor in the 2014 American College of Cardiology/American Heart Association[59] guidelines. A study of 564,267 outpatient surgical procedures demonstrated that along with advancing age (>85 years), factors for postoperative mortality included invasiveness of the surgical procedures and the need for hospitalization.[48] Many other studies have shown a similar association after noncardiac surgery with a high ASA score,[46,50] invasiveness of the surgical procedure,[49,50,60] as well as advancing age. Within an older population, emergency surgery and wait time for emergency surgery are known risk factors for adverse outcomes.[4,49,50,53,61,62] Another study showed that older adults with ischemic and nonischemic heart failure are at higher risk of postoperative mortality (9%) than older adults with coronary artery disease (3%) after a noncardiac surgery.[53]

Although clinical outcomes research is the most common type of research conducted in anesthesia, there is a scarcity of studies looking at high-risk factors, specifically within the geriatric population. Most of the information related to the geriatric population is derived from studies that include all adults with subgroup analyses on the older cohort. It is essential to identify specific risk factors in the geriatric population that can help risk stratify them and, thereby, help formulate individualized perioperative care plans for high-risk patients.

Application of Machine and Deep Learning Tools

In the last decade, there has been an exponential increase in the application of machine learning (ML)[63] and deep learning (DL) tools in medicine.[64] Many studies have emerged showing the utility and efficacy of ML/DL tools in different aspects of anesthesia and perioperative care.[65,66] In a systematic review, 35 studies were identified that illustrated the efficacy of specific ML/DL tools in predicting postsurgical outcomes such as pain, sepsis, intensive care unit (ICU) admission, acute kidney injury, mortality, and various neurological, respiratory, and cardiovascular complications.[66] These predictors are significant in the setting of the geriatric population, where such complications can have catastrophic effects. Another utility of ML/DL is the control of anesthesia and drug delivery. Intraoperatively, older adults are associated with rapid and unpredictable physiological and pharmacological demands. Control systems with feedforward and feedback systems can automate the delivery of anesthesia and neuromuscular blockade.[67] Continuous metrics such as blood pressure, electroencephalogram, bispectral index, and physiological parameters have been used to determine anesthesia needs.[68–70] Advances in ML/DL tools can forecast drug pharmacokinetics to provide accurate delivery of paralytics[71] in a high-risk population. ML/DL tools can also be integrated in ultrasound-guided techniques.[65] Optimal vascular or epidural access for the elderly patient remains a challenge.[72] Recently, studies have emerged demonstrating neural networks can be used to identify vascular structures such as femoral artery while distinguishing similar-appearing ultrasound images.[73] Additionally, other studies have demonstrated an accuracy of up to 95% in determining important spine column structures in real time,[74,75] techniques which help reduce error while approaching invasive procedures in the geriatric patient.

Briefly, tools such as gradient boosting, logistic regression, random forest, support vector, decision tree, k-nearest, neural networks such as convolutional neural networks, and reinforcement learning are already actively used in perioperative research.[66] Because of open-source initiatives by the industry, most ML/DL tools are free and come with tremendous community support, making them lucrative research tools to advance geriatric perioperative care.

Wearable Devices

The introduction of advanced electronic wearable devices has helped us record continuous, high-quality physiological measures that were not previously possible. These devices are currently being used to monitor physiological parameters continuously in the general population, detect arrhythmia,[76] and optimize training in athletes.[77] The concept of continuously monitoring vitals was recently used by Eddahchouri and colleagues.[78] In this study, continuous monitoring of patient vital signs using wearable monitoring technology was associated with a reduction in unplanned ICU admissions and rapid response team calls. This is one of many emerging studies demonstrating the usefulness of wearable devices.[79] These devices have become a vital source of rich data that can be fed to powerful ML algorithms to understand each patient better and tailor treatments accordingly. For example, the physiological data including heart rate, resting heart rate, heart rate variability, skin temperature, and blood oxygen levels from wearable devices are currently being used to provide recommendations to optimize athletic performance.[80] A similar approach can be taken to optimize physiology in older patients before an elective procedure. Continuous physiological and accelerometer data can also be used to determine which patients are at an increased risk of postoperative delirium or arrhythmias.[79,81] Another potential application of wearable devices can be to reduce alarm fatigue.[79] Alarm fatigue is defined as sensory overload when health-care providers are exposed to multiple alarms, which can cause desensitization and subsequently, lead to missed alarms.[82] Continuous monitoring using a wearable device can establish intrasubject variability in the physiological data and characterize the alarm's threshold and prioritization of alarms at an individual level.[79] This application can be beneficial while taking care of older adults who usually present with abnormal physiological baselines.

Visual Analytics

Attributes of big data include velocity (data generated at high speed), volume (large size), and variety (diversity)[32]; therefore, big data pose computing challenges. The usage of big data is limited because it may require specialized skill sets to handle the data. Visual analytics (VA) can be an optimal solution that can help generalize the usage and unlock big data's full potential. VA tools provide sophisticated computing tools integrated with visual interfaces with the ability to interact and manipulate data in real time.[83,84] Thus, providing solutions such as point-and-click exploration instead of manually writing queries, a more comprehensive visual review of the data and results using graphs, and displaying large amounts of filtered data in simpler forms.[85,86]

VA can be applied to health-care and research data in the fields of genomics and epidemiology. VAs are currently used in select institutions to aid clinical operations. Examples include dashboards to monitor symptom evolution during disease progression,[87] performing pharmacokinetic–pharmacodynamic analyses,[88] and visualizing outcomes data.[89] In the setting of continuously improving electronic health records and anesthesia information management systems (AIMS), VA can offer promising tools to leverage data to improve perioperative care and enhance health-care education,[90] therefore, bridging the gap between the medical and data sciences.[91]

RESEARCH CONSIDERATIONS

There is an enormous amount of data and numerous questions that can be answered with these datasets. However, it is essential to follow a systematic path to provide meaningful results. Some general considerations include the following: first, to decide the aim of the study—what is the question?—and check whether an appropriate dataset is available to answer this question. Second, assess the quality of data. Are the data complete and consistent? Have the data been internally or externally verified for the key variables? Incomplete data do not preclude a study; however, they may introduce biases, especially when key variables and prognostic variables of interest are missing.[92] It is important to remember that missing data do not represent the absence or presence of a variable and should be considered accordingly.[93] Third, is the eligible population captured adequately? Are the data representative of the population of interest? For example, if looking at patients aged older than 65 years undergoing hip surgeries using a state dataset, it is essential to confirm whether the subselected population is similar to national averages. Fourth, does the analysis account for critical variables and cofounders that may influence outcomes? Fifth, are the inferences and conclusions justified and generalizable? Moreover, if causal interpretation is provided, it is vital to provide alternate explanations. No matter how big data are or how complicated analyses are, it is always important to follow the basic principles of statistical reporting in an effort to provide accurate results.

CHALLENGES

Big data can come with big problems. Decreased enrollment and reduced retention of older adults is the biggest challenge faced in big data research. Barriers to recruitment include significant health problems, knowledge gaps, social and cultural barriers, and incapacity to provide informed consent. Recruitment is more challenging in institutionalized and hospitalized older patients, adding another layer of complexity to geriatric research. Mody and colleagues[94] report fundamental approaches that maximize recruitment include timely screening and identification, in-depth explanation of the study, minimizing exclusion criteria, securing the cooperation of all parties involved such as nursing facilities. In addition, providing incremental incentives, continued communication, carefully reviewing the study's overall progress, targeting specific strategies to the condition and population of interest, anticipating potential problems, and promptly employing contingency plans are keys to effective retention.[94] Implementation cost is a considerable challenge in adopting big data research. The hospitals and clinics must hire skilled personnel and acquire specialized computational and custom applications for data collection. Although large academic institutions can afford this infrastructure and gather valuable data, smaller community and rural hospitals may need help adopting big data solutions. In the context of geriatric population research, this difference alone can create bias because an older population with care established at small local hospitals may not be included in national-level studies. Privacy and data security are integral parts of data science. Data breaches are common in all industries, especially health care. Decreased focus on data security makes medical research data most vulnerable to breaches. Patient specific identity information from health-care and research databases can be misused especially in older adults who are commonly targeted for fraudulent schemes. According to a recent report in

2021, US$239 million in losses were suffered by people aged 60 years and older in various investment scams. This highlights the paramount importance of data security especially in dealing with a vulnerable population such as the older adults.

SUMMARY

Future of anesthesia research needs to focus on the older adults. The elderly population undergoes a disproportionately higher number of surgeries and the prevalence of anesthetic encounters in this population is steadily increasing. Big data provides a unique opportunity in providing information that can advance perioperative care in elderly. Using sophisticated tools and skill sets that are now commonly available, we can understand the complex nature of geriatric anesthesia and aid the providers taking care of older adults in routine clinical decision-making. Although we promote big data research, it is important to recognize unique challenges that are faced by this vulnerable population and cater our solutions accordingly.

CLINICS CARE POINTS

- The proportion of the older patients undergoing surgeries has increased, leading to increasing interest in geriatric anesthesiology.
- Large sample sizes and diverse elderly populations captured by large nationwide datasets can provide robust evidence for better geriatric perioperative care.
- Promoting collaboration and data sharing between institutions will encourage big data research in geriatric anesthesiology.
- Sophisticated tools, such as machine learning and deep learning, can make precision medicine for the older population a reality.

CONFLICTS OF INTEREST AND SOURCES OF FUNDING

Dr A. Bardia is supported by the R01 HS029172-01 grant by the Agency for Healthcare Research and Quality (AHRQ), United States. None of the authors has any conflicts of interest.

REFERENCES

1. Postoperative delirium in older adults: best practice statement from the American Geriatrics Society. J Am Coll Surg 2015;220(2):136–48.e1.
2. Deiner S. Adherence to recommended practices for perioperative anesthesia care for older adults among US anesthesiologists: results from the ASA Committee on Geriatric Anesthesia-Perioperative Brain Health Initiative ASA member survey. Perioperat Med 2020;9(1):6.
3. Cullen KA, Hall MJ, Golosinskiy A. Ambulatory surgery in the United States, 2006. Natl Health Stat Report 2009;(11):1–25.
4. Turrentine FE. Surgical risk factors, morbidity, and mortality in elderly patients. J Am Coll Surg 2006;203(6):865–77.
5. Hood R. Peri-operative neurological complications. Anaesthesia 2018;73(S1): 67–75.
6. Cadarette SM, Wong L. An introduction to health care administrative data. Can J Hosp Pharm 2015;68(3):232–7.

7. AHRQ. Available at: http://www.qualityindicators.ahrq.gov/downloads/modules/psi/v30/psi_technical_specs_v30.pdf. Accessed September 2, 2022.

8. Agency for Healthcare Research and Quality. R., MD. HCUP Overview. Healthcare Cost and Utilization Project (HCUP). 2022. Available at: www.hcup-us.ahrq.gov/overview.jsp. Accessed September 2, 2022.

9. Nassar AK. Virtual reality (VR) as a simulation modality for technical skills acquisition. Ann Med Surg (Lond) 2021;71:102945.

10. Liu J. Hospital-based acute care within 7 days of discharge after outpatient arthroscopic shoulder surgery. Anesth Analg 2018;126(2):600–5.

11. Banco D. Perioperative cardiovascular outcomes among older adults undergoing in-hospital noncardiac surgery. J Am Geriatr Soc 2021;69(10):2821–30.

12. Rubin DS. Local anesthetic systemic toxicity in total joint arthroplasty: incidence and risk factors in the United States from the national inpatient sample 1998-2013. Reg Anesth Pain Med 2018;43(2):131–7.

13. Premier Applied Sciences®, P.I. Premier Healthcare Database White Paper: Data that informs and performs. March 2, 2020. Available at: https://products.premierinc.com/downloads/PremierHealthcareDatabaseWhitepaper.pdf. Accessed April 8, 2023.

14. Zhong H. An overview of commonly used data sources in observational research in anesthesia. Anesth Analg 2022;134(3):548–58.

15. Wasserman I. Impact of intravenous acetaminophen on perioperative opioid utilization and outcomes in open colectomies: a claims database analysis. Anesthesiology 2018;129(1):77–88.

16. Stundner O. Effectiveness of intravenous acetaminophen for postoperative pain management in hip and knee arthroplasties: a population-based study. Reg Anesth Pain Med 2019;44(5):565–72.

17. Mörwald EE. Intravenous acetaminophen does not reduce inpatient opioid prescription or opioid-related adverse events among patients undergoing spine surgery. Anesth Analg 2018;127(5):1221–8.

18. Memtsoudis S. Risk factors for postoperative delirium in patients undergoing lower extremity joint arthroplasty: a retrospective population-based cohort study. Regional Anesthesia & Pain Medicine 2019;44(10):934.

19. Kulaylat AS. Truven health analytics marketscan databases for clinical research in colon and rectal surgery. Clin Colon Rectal Surg 2019;32(1):54–60.

20. McIsaac DI. Association of polypharmacy with survival, complications, and healthcare resource use after elective noncardiac surgery: a population-based cohort study. Anesthesiology 2018;128(6):1140–50.

21. McIsaac DI. The association of frailty with outcomes and resource use after emergency general surgery: a population-based cohort study. Anesth Analg 2017;124(5):1653–61.

22. Wilson L. Risk factors for new-onset depression or anxiety following total joint arthroplasty: the role of chronic opioid use. Regional Anesthesia & Pain Medicine 2019;44(11):990.

23. Ladha KS. Impact of perioperative epidural placement on postdischarge opioid use in patients undergoing abdominal surgery. Anesthesiology 2016;124(2):396–403.

24. Steinberg SM. Comparison of risk adjustment methodologies in surgical quality improvement. Surgery 2008;144(4):662–7 [discussion: 662-7].

25. Bellomy ML. The attributable mortality of postoperative bleeding exceeds the attributable mortality of postoperative venous thromboembolism. Anesth Analg 2021;132(1):82–8.

26. Brovman EY. Anesthesia type is not associated with postoperative complications in the care of patients with lower extremity traumatic fractures. Anesth Analg 2019;129(4):1034–42.

27. Kim EM, Li G, Kim M. Development of a risk score to predict postoperative delirium in patients with hip fracture. Anesth Analg 2020;130(1):79–86.

28. Liau A. The national anesthesia clinical outcomes registry. Anesth Analg 2015; 121(6):1604–10.

29. Lam S. Trends in peripheral nerve block usage in mastectomy and lumpectomy: analysis of a national database from 2010 to 2018. Anesth Analg 2021;133(1): 32–40.

30. Gabriel RA. The patterns of utilization of interscalene nerve blocks for total shoulder arthroplasty. Anesth Analg 2016;123(3):758–61.

31. Glance LG. Variability in case durations for common surgical procedures. Anesth Analg 2018;126(6):2017–24.

32. Levin MA, Wanderer JP, Ehrenfeld JM. Data, big data, and metadata in anesthesiology. Anesth Analg 2015;121(6):1661–7.

33. Aziz MF. Success of intubation rescue techniques after failed direct laryngoscopy in adults: a retrospective comparative analysis from the multicenter perioperative outcomes group. Anesthesiology 2016;125(4):656–66.

34. Berman MF. Alarm limits for intraoperative drug infusions: a report from the multicenter perioperative outcomes group. Anesth Analg 2017;125(4):1203–11.

35. Colquhoun DA. A lower tidal volume regimen during one-lung ventilation for lung resection surgery is not associated with reduced postoperative pulmonary complications. Anesthesiology 2021;134(4):562–76.

36. Villa G, Romagnoli S. Registers and biobanks in ICU and anesthesia. Minerva Anestesiol 2022;88(10):864–9.

37. Tigchelaar C. The Anaesthetic Biobank of Cerebrospinal fluid: a unique repository for neuroscientific biomarker research. Ann Transl Med 2021;9(6):455.

38. Kroma RB. Implementation of the uniformed services university pain registry biobank: a military and veteran population–focused biobank and registry. Pain Med 2021;22(12):2950–63.

39. Fried LP. Frailty in older adults: evidence for a phenotype. J Gerontol A Biol Sci Med Sci 2001;56(3):M146–56.

40. Clegg A. Frailty in elderly people. Lancet 2013;381(9868):752–62.

41. Collard RM. Prevalence of frailty in community-dwelling older persons: a systematic review. J Am Geriatr Soc 2012;60(8):1487–92.

42. Hubbard RE, Story DA. Does frailty lie in the eyes of the beholder? Heart Lung Circ 2015;24(6):525–6.

43. Lee J. Modified frailty index predicts postoperative complications following panniculectomy in the elderly. Plastic and Reconstructive Surgery – Global Open 2020;8(7):e2987.

44. Chang CM. Adjusted age-adjusted charlson comorbidity index score as a risk measure of perioperative mortality before cancer surgery. PLoS One 2016; 11(2):e0148076.

45. Chow WB. Optimal preoperative assessment of the geriatric surgical patient: a best practices guideline from the American College of Surgeons National Surgical Quality Improvement Program and the American Geriatrics Society. J Am Coll Surg 2012;215(4):453–66.

46. Hamel MB. Surgical outcomes for patients aged 80 and older: morbidity and mortality from major noncardiac surgery. J Am Geriatr Soc 2005;53(3):424–9.

47. Kheterpal S. Preoperative and intraoperative predictors of cardiac adverse events after general, vascular, and urological surgery. Anesthesiology 2009; 110(1):58–66.
48. Fleisher LA. Inpatient hospital admission and death after outpatient surgery in elderly patients: importance of patient and system characteristics and location of care. Arch Surg 2004;139(1):67–72.
49. Pedersen T, Eliasen K, Henriksen E. A prospective study of mortality associated with anaesthesia and surgery: risk indicators of mortality in hospital. Acta Anaesthesiol Scand 1990;34(3):176–82.
50. Hosking MP. Outcomes of surgery in patients 90 years of age and older. JAMA 1989;261(13):1909–15.
51. Chung F, Mezei G, Tong D. Adverse events in ambulatory surgery. A comparison between elderly and younger patients. Can J Anaesth 1999;46(4):309–21.
52. Smetana GW, Lawrence VA, Cornell JE. Preoperative pulmonary risk stratification for noncardiothoracic surgery: systematic review for the American College of Physicians. Ann Intern Med 2006;144(8):581–95.
53. van Diepen S. Mortality and readmission of patients with heart failure, atrial fibrillation, or coronary artery disease undergoing noncardiac surgery: an analysis of 38 047 patients. Circulation 2011;124(3):289–96.
54. Hammill BG. Impact of heart failure on patients undergoing major noncardiac surgery. Anesthesiology 2008;108(4):559–67.
55. Kheterpal S. Development and validation of an acute kidney injury risk index for patients undergoing general surgery: results from a national data set. Anesthesiology 2009;110(3):505–15.
56. Evered LA, Silbert BS. Postoperative cognitive dysfunction and noncardiac surgery. Anesth Analg 2018;127(2):496–505.
57. Helen OB. Mind over matter? The hidden epidemic of cognitive dysfunction in the older surgical patient. Ann Surg 2017;265(4):677–91.
58. Saczynski JS. Cognitive trajectories after postoperative delirium. N Engl J Med 2012;367(1):30–9.
59. Fleisher LA. 2014 ACC/AHA guideline on perioperative cardiovascular evaluation and management of patients undergoing noncardiac surgery: executive summary: a report of the American College of Cardiology/American Heart Association Task Force on Practice Guidelines. Circulation 2014;130(24):2215–45.
60. Balentine CJ. Postacute Care after major abdominal surgery in elderly patients: intersection of age, functional status, and postoperative complications. JAMA Surg 2016;151(8):759–66.
61. Liu LL, Leung JM. Predicting adverse postoperative outcomes in patients aged 80 years or older. J Am Geriatr Soc 2000;48(4):405–12.
62. Pincus D. Association between wait time and 30-day mortality in adults undergoing hip fracture surgery. JAMA 2017;318(20):1994–2003.
63. Winkler P. Short video interventions to reduce mental health stigma: a multi-centre randomised controlled trial in nursing high schools. Soc Psychiatry Psychiatr Epidemiol 2017;52(12):1549–57.
64. Rajkomar A, Dean J, Kohane I. Machine learning in medicine. N Engl J Med 2019; 380(14):1347–58.
65. Hashimoto DA. Artificial intelligence in anesthesiology: current techniques, clinical applications, and limitations. Anesthesiology 2020;132(2):379–94.
66. Bellini V. Machine learning in perioperative medicine: a systematic review. Journal of Anesthesia, Analgesia and Critical Care 2022;2(1):2.

67. Dumont GA, Ansermino JM. Closed-loop control of anesthesia: a primer for anesthesiologists. Anesth Analg 2013;117(5):1130–8.
68. Tsutsui T, Arita S. Fuzzy-logic control of blood pressure through enflurane anesthesia. J Clin Monit 1994;10(2):110–7.
69. Zbinden AM. Arterial pressure control with isoflurane using fuzzy logic. Br J Addiction: Br J Anaesth 1995;74(1):66–72.
70. Absalom AR, Sutcliffe N, Kenny GN. Closed-loop control of anesthesia using bispectral index: performance assessment in patients undergoing major orthopedic surgery under combined general and regional anesthesia. The Journal of the American Society of Anesthesiologists 2002;96(1):67–73.
71. Motamed C. Influence of real-time Bayesian forecasting of pharmacokinetic parameters on the precision of a rocuronium target-controlled infusion. Eur J Clin Pharmacol 2012;68(7):1025–31.
72. Gabriel J. Understanding the challenges to vascular access in an ageing population. Br J Nurs 2017;26(14):S15–23.
73. Smistad E, Løvstakken L. Vessel detection in ultrasound images using deep convolutional neural networks. In: Deep learning and data labeling for medical applications. Springer; 2016. p. 30–8. Available at: https://www.eriksmistad.no/upload/Vessel_detection_in_ultrasound_images_using_deep_convolutional_neural_networks_Preprint.pdf. Accessed April 8, 2023.
74. Hetherington J. SLIDE: automatic spine level identification system using a deep convolutional neural network. Int J Comput Assist Radiol Surg 2017;12(7):1189–98.
75. Pesteie M. Automatic localization of the needle target for ultrasound-guided epidural injections. IEEE Trans Med Imaging 2017;37(1):81–92.
76. Cheung CC, Krahn AD, Andrade JG. The emerging role of wearable technologies in detection of arrhythmia. Can J Cardiol 2018;34(8):1083–7.
77. Bellenger CR, Miller D, Halson SL, et al. Evaluating the Typical Day-to-Day Variability of WHOOP-Derived Heart Rate Variability in Olympic Water Polo Athletes. Sensors (Basel) 2022;22(18):6723.
78. Eddahchouri Y. Effect of continuous wireless vital sign monitoring on unplanned ICU admissions and rapid response team calls: a before-and-after study. Br J Anaesth 2022;128(5):857–63.
79. Webster CS, Scheeren TWL, Wan YI. Patient monitoring, wearable devices, and the healthcare information ecosystem. Br J Anaesth 2022;128(5):756–8.
80. Miller DJ, Sargent C, Roach GD. A Validation of Six Wearable Devices for Estimating Sleep, Heart Rate and Heart Rate Variability in Healthy Adults. Sensors (Basel) 2022;22(16):6317.
81. Davoudi A. Role of wearable accelerometer devices in delirium studies: a systematic review. Crit Care Explor 2019;1(9):e0027.
82. Sendelbach S, Funk M. Alarm fatigue: a patient safety concern. AACN Adv Crit Care 2013;24(4):378–86 [quiz: 387-8].
83. Simpao AF. A review of analytics and clinical informatics in health care. J Med Syst 2014;38(4):45.
84. Gillespie G. Getting a visual on health analytics. Health Data Manag 2014;22(7):39–42.
85. Youn-Ah K, Görg C, Stasko J. How can visual analytics assist investigative analysis? design implications from an evaluation. IEEE Trans Vis Comput Graph 2011;17(5):570–83.
86. Ola O, Sedig K. The challenge of big data in public health: an opportunity for visual analytics. Online J Public Health Inform 2014;5(3):223.

87. Perer A, Sun J. MatrixFlow: temporal network visual analytics to track symptom evolution during disease progression. AMIA Annu Symp Proc 2012;2012:716–25.
88. Goldsmith MR. PAVA: physiological and anatomical visual analytics for mapping of tissue-specific concentration and time-course data. J Pharmacokinet Pharmacodyn 2010;37(3):277–87.
89. Rajwan YG. Visualizing central line -associated blood stream infection (CLABSI) outcome data for decision making by health care consumers and practitioners-an evaluation study. Online J Public Health Inform 2013;5(2):218.
90. Vaitsis C, Nilsson G, Zary N. Big data in medical informatics: improving education through visual analytics. Stud Health Technol Inform 2014;205:1163–7.
91. Simpao AF, Ahumada LM, Rehman MA. Big data and visual analytics in anaesthesia and health care†. Br J Addiction: Br J Anaesth 2015;115(3):350–6.
92. Howe CJ, Cain LE, Hogan JW. Are all biases missing data problems? Curr Epidemiol Rep 2015;2(3):162–71.
93. Dong Y, Peng CY. Principled missing data methods for researchers. SpringerPlus 2013;2(1):222.
94. Mody L. Recruitment and retention of older adults in aging research. J Am Geriatr Soc 2008;56(12):2340–8.

Enhanced Recovery After Surgery and Elderly Patients
Advances

Olle Ljungqvist, MD, PhD[a],*, Hans D. de Boer, MD, PhD[b]

KEYWORDS

- Surgery • Anesthesia • Recovery • Older patients • Frailty • Complications • ERAS

KEY POINTS

- Enhanced recovery after surgery (ERAS) care minimizes the stress of surgery.
- Older frail risk patients recover better from surgery with ERAS.
- The reduction of stress with ERAS is likely to benefit this patient group.

INTRODUCTION AND A BRIEF HISTORY

Enhanced recovery after surgery (ERAS) represents a specific approach to the care of the surgical patient. ERAS entails a perioperative care protocol based on care elements with scientific evidence of supporting recovery and reducing complications. ERAS involves all caregivers and stakeholders involved in the surgery. From the caregivers, a local ERAS team is formed including the doctors, nurses, nutritionists, physiotherapists, and other allied health professionals from all specialties and units involved. The ERAS team remains in close contact with the management of the hospital, while involving and engaging the patient and their immediate close ones at the center of the care. A key aspect of ERAS is that the care delivery is kept under control by continuous audit and feedback of how well the caregivers follow the ERAS Guidelines and the outcomes of their care with regard to recoveries and complications.

The ideas and concepts of ERAS were founded by a group of surgeons from the Northern parts of Europe early this century.[1] A little more than 20 years ago, Kenneth Fearon from Edinburgh met with Olle Ljungqvist from Stockholm and together they invited colleagues and their teams from Norway (Arthur Revhaug, Tromsö), Denmark (Henrik Kehlet, Copenhagen), and The Netherlands (Martin von Meyenfeldt, Maastricht)

[a] Department of Surgery, School of Medical Sciences, Örebro University, Orebro SE-701 85, Sweden; [b] Department of Anesthesia, Pain Medicine and Procedural Sedation and Analgesia, Martini General Hospital Groningen, Van Swietenplein 1, 9728 NT, Groningen, the Netherlands
* Corresponding author.
E-mail address: olle.ljungqvist@oru.se

Anesthesiology Clin 41 (2023) 647–655
https://doi.org/10.1016/j.anclin.2023.02.010
1932-2275/23/© 2023 Elsevier Inc. All rights reserved.
anesthesiology.theclinics.com

to initiate a program to set up a guidance for best practice in colonic resections. The group was very much inspired by the study of Henrik Kehlet who had popularized the multimodal approach to recovery after surgery with his Fast Track concept.[2,3] The ERAS Study Group (as they named themselves) set out to take these ideas one step further. They decided to review the literature to seek care items that would support the recovery of the patient. Based on their findings, they published the first consensus article on ERAS in 2005.[4] This was the first time that a perioperative guide, which included care elements identified to improve outcomes and reviewed for their efficacy, was assembled in a standardized way.

Later studies proved this approach, to use the knowledge available in the medical literature and assemble them to a care protocol care, to be very successful. Large patient series showed repeatedly an association between better compliance to the guideline elements and shorter stay, fewer complications, and readmissions.[5–7] The articles of short-term outcomes were later followed by reports, finding improved long-term survival with higher guideline adherence.[8] The short-term outcomes have since been confirmed in many studies around the world and for different specialties,[9,10] and available long-term outcomes tend to show positive outcomes with either no difference in survival or improved survival being reported.[10] There were a few other important breakthroughs that led to the formal start of the ERAS Society (www.erassociety.org) in 2010 from the ERAS Study Group. By 2010, it was clear from the literature that ERAS protocols would have a major impact on the improving outcomes. A meta-analysis of several randomized trials showed an almost 50% reduction in complications with ERAS protocols compared with traditional care.[11] The change from impact mainly in shortening length of stay to a substantial reduction in complications raised the interest considerably among colleagues around the world. The Dutch colleagues under the leadership of Cornelius DeJong and Jose Maassen working with the Kwaliteitsinstituut in the Netherlands reported that after 10 months of implementation training of the ERAS guidelines, hospital stay could be brought down by at least 30% and often more.[12] With the growing information of its potential and subsequent interest in ERAS, the group decided to form the ERAS Society in 2010.[1]

This review explains the basis for ERAS from the point of view of its founding organization, how it works, and why it works and focusses especially on the impact it may have in the elderly population undergoing surgery.

MECHANISMS BEHIND THE RESULTS OF ENHANCED RECOVERY AFTER SURGERY

The basis for the effects of the ERAS protocols lies with the mode of action of its individual care components. When reviewing their individual effects on the body, most ERAS care items either reduce the stress of the injury caused by the operation or help avoid unnecessary side effects (**Table 1**).[13] The reduction of stress and the burden it places on vulnerable organs with limited resilience becomes especially important for the patient who may be compromised to start with by frailty,[14] or concomitant disease,[15,16] that are often present in the elderly populations.

THE ENHANCED RECOVERY AFTER SURGERY GUIDELINES—SPREADING ACROSS SURGERY

Since the publication of the first consensus guidelines for, colonic resection in 2005, the ERAS Society has published guidelines in collaboration with experts around the globe for almost all major operations (**Table 2**), and more are in the making and revisions and updates are made as needed (www.erassociety.org)[17]. Although the initial article was a consensus by a group of academic surgeons with decades of

Table 1
Enhanced recovery after surgery care items and their principal mode of action to support recovery and avoid complications

ERAS Care Items	Mode of Main Action in Support of Recovery
Preadmission items	
Smoke cessation	Reduce complications
Alcohol cessation	Reduce complications
Nutrition care for undernourished	Reduce complications
Immunonutrition	Reduce postoperative infections
Prehabilitation	Improve stress resilience, support postoperative mobility
Preoperative items	
Avoiding bowel preparation	Avoid fluid balance disturbances
Preoperative carbohydrate drink	Help maintain control of glucose, retain muscle mass and function
Preoperative antibiotic prophylaxis	Reduce infectious complications
Preoperative thrombosis prophylaxis	Minimize risk of postoperative thrombosis
Intraoperative items	
Fluid balance	Maintaining fluid balance, avoiding overload and dehydration Support gut motility
Regional anesthesia	Reducing long-acting opioid use in support of gut motility Avoiding post operative nausea and vomiting (PONV)
Minimal invasive surgery	Reduce inflammatory response and pain Support return of gut movements
Balanced multimodal analgesia	Reduce the use of long-acting opioid use
Postoperative items	
Early oral feeding	Avoid long time fasting, stimulate gut motility, provide energy and protein
Early mobilization	Stimulate normal behavior as soon as possible, strengthen muscles
Multimodal pain management	Avoid side effects of opioid use for gut motility and support mobility Minimize the risk of opioid-induced PONV

experience in clinical research, the processes of producing these guidelines have been refined over the years as described in a recent publication.[18] Currently, the GRADE system is used as the basis for the guidelines, and evidence is graded in a systematic way giving the reader a full insight to how strong the science is for any given care item. This is coupled with a recommendation for its use with either a weak or a strong recommendation also considering the effectiveness of treatments and potential risks of harm and if the group feels that new data would have a chance to change the recommendation (weak) or not (strong). What has been revealed when performing this study is that many types of operations do not have data from that specific surgery as the basis for a given recommendation. There have simply not been any studies performed in that specific operation to address the use of some care elements, and information from similar operations must be used as a surrogate.

Table 2
Enhanced recovery after surgery society guidelines latest versions as of 2022

Area of Surgery	Authors	Journal and Year
Abdominal surgery LMIC	Oodit R et al	World J Surg 2022
Bariatric surgery	Stenberg E et al World	J Surg 2022
Open aortic surgery	McGringle KL et al	J Vasc Surg 2022
Spine surgery	DeBono et al	Spine J 2021
Emergency laparotomy 1	Peden C et al	World J Surg 2021
Hip and knee replacement	Wainwright T et al	Acta Orthop 2020
Pancreatoduodenectomy	Melloul E et al	World J Surg 2020
Neonatal intestinal surgery	Brindle M et al	World J Surg 2020
HIPEC part 1	Hübner M et al	Eur J Surg Oncol 2020
HIPEC part 2	Hübner M et al	Eur J Surg Oncol 2020
Vulvar and vaginal surgery	Altman AD	Am J Obstet Gynecol 2020
Esophagectomy	Low DE et al	World J Surg 2019
Gynecologic oncology	Nelson G et al	Int J Gyn Cancer 2019
Lung surgery	Batchelor T et al	Eur J Cardiothor Surg 2019
Cardiac surgery	Engelman DT et al	JAMA Surg 2019
Colorectal surgery	Gustafsson U et al	World J Surg 2018
Caeserean Section part 1	Wilson RD et al	Am J Obstet Gynecol 2018
Caeserean Section part 2	Wilson RD et al	Am J Obstet Gynecol 2018
Caeserean Section part 3	Macones GA et al	Am J Obstet Gynecol 2018
Breast reconstruction	Temple-Oberle C et al	Plastb Recon Surg 2017
Head and neck cancer surgery	Dort J et al JAMA	Otol head neck 2017
Anesthesia practice	Feldheiser A et al	Acta Anaesth Scand 2017
Liver resection	Melloul E et al	World J Surg 2016
Gastrectomy	Mortensen K et al	Br J Surg 2014
Cystectomy	Certantola Y et al	Clin Nutr 2013

All the latest guidelines are available at the ERAS Society website: www.erassociety.org.

WHY ENHANCED RECOVERY AFTER SURGERY HAS BECOME THE FOCUS IN SURGERY AND ANESTHESIA?

The reason ERAS programs have become so popular is that they deliver the results all stakeholders aim for. Patients recover quicker, have fewer complications, go back to normal activities faster including back to work, and long-term outcomes suggest better survival after cancer surgery. Health-care professionals see the effect of ERAS with their own eyes daily. Patients can eat and drink while mobilizing much faster than with traditional care. Surgeons find patients experiencing fewer and less severe complications and find less use of intensive care unit (ICU) support. Pain teams see less side effects of pain medication, and nurses and Allied Health Professionals find their patients return to activities much faster. Hospital managers are finding more space available on wards and ICU, allowing for more patient throughput, and while avoiding costly reoperations, intensive care, and readmissions.[19–21] These factors also help build the reputation of the hospital with additional positive impact on referrals and revenue. Finally, society and the general public is saving costs for health care, not only by the above effects on in-hospital care but also for less use of health-care facilities once discharged from the hospital, and fewer days off from work and contributing to the society in a more general sense. Although the clinical effects of the ERAS program were first evident in major colorectal surgery, since then many specialties have reported similar gains—reductions in length of stay, fewer complications, and lower cost.[17]

EXPERIENCES IN MAKING ENHANCED RECOVERY AFTER SURGERY WORK IN PRACTICE

The guidelines discuss all elements of care from before the patient is admitted to a follow-up at least 30 days after surgery. Because all professions contribute to the care of the patient during her/his journey, it is essential that every profession is represented in running the ERAS care pathway. This is arranged by setting up a local ERAS team that is led by the 3 main professions and specialties—surgery, anesthesia, and nursing. The ERAS Society has developed an ERAS Implementation Program based on building a local ERAS team around this trio of health-care professionals.[22] This team is complemented by representatives from all areas that the patient passes through in the perioperative period and all professionals groups involved. Because this team will have to have dedicated and protected time for this teamwork 1 hour or so every 2 to 4 weeks, management support is essential to make this work. In addition, the nurse is usually given the task to do much of the day-to-day running of the program and to collect data for audit (see later discussion). Moreover, for reasons explained above this is probably one of the best investments that can be made in the perioperative medicine today.

The team needs to get control over the care in the institution. This is achieved by collecting data on care processes and outcomes in a standardized way and using this for continuous audit. The ERAS Society has helped institutions in more than 30 countries around the world to implement ERAS. During this work, it has consistently been our experience that very rarely someone is in full control of what is going on, and so far in all the training performed by the ERAS Society, no single unit have been correct in their belief of what is being done to their patients at the level needed to get control. By auditing, the team and everyone in the departments can, usually for the first time, see the details of the care being delivered with insights to what is functioning and what may be failing delivery. This is the starting point for initiating the drive of change toward a higher compliance with the guidelines. For most units the starting point is typically around $50 \pm 10\%$ compliance to the guidelines. It is common that several guideline elements are missing, although some are in use but with inconsistency. These care elements can be targeted for implementation or improved consistency, to result in better care. Usually, the teams learn how to drive change during a period of 3 to 4 months and then spend another 4 to 5 months to fine tune their ERAS care to reach a level of compliance above 70%, which typically results in better outcomes.[5]

ENHANCED RECOVERY AFTER SURGERY AND THE ELDERLY

During the last several decades, the age when a patient was considered fit enough for surgery has been raised considerably because the age expectancy has increased. Today chronological age is less of a factor, and patients in their 90s and older are operated worldwide. Still, elderly patients need longer to recover from major surgery,[2] have a higher risk of perioperative complications and increased morbidity and mortality, mostly as result of their comorbidities and decreased physiological reserve capacity.[14–16]

Moreover, frailty is a common clinical condition with increasing age and represents a major contributing factor in increasing the risk for a poor outcome of surgical care in this patient population.[14] Although frailty is more common with older age, it can also be present in younger patients. For the surgical patient, it is important to realize that frailty represents a global risk state and not a fixed diagnosis. The main contributors to frailty are poor physical performance, poor cognition, malnutrition, and poor mental health.[14] In different combinations, these factors lead to deficits that affect outcomes in surgery including comorbidities, poor nutrition intake, weight and muscle loss, weakness, and physical decline that all increase the risk of complications and the recovery after operations.

As stated above, there is clear evidence from several surgical specialties that implementation of ERAS care results in a reduction of complications, improved outcome and is associated with increased survival compared with non-ERAS or more traditional care. Therefore, it was likely that ERAS protocols would be beneficial in the perioperative care also in elderly patients, and reports already at the very start of the era of Fast Track/ERAS more than 20 years ago suggested this to be the case.[2,23]

The increasing literature in elderly patients undergoing ERAS care shows evidence that this patient population benefit from ERAS.[24–26] However, there are also limitations in interpretation of the existing data as result of variation in existing ERAS protocols in place and the large variation of comorbidities in the patient population studied.[24–26]

Several database studies in colorectal surgery report that elderly patients treated according to ERAS principles had slightly more cardiovascular complications compared with younger patients (10% vs 4%) but overall, older patients do not suffer from serious complications more often than younger patients.[27] In general, in ERAS settings, the overall complication rate is reported to be low in the elderly (above 70 years of age) and similar to those reported from patients aged younger than 70 years of age.[24–27] Furthermore, in these database studies in the high-risk elderly patients, the time to return to normal daily living was slightly increased as was the length of hospital stay compared with younger patients. A retrospective study in laparoscopic colorectal surgery studied how well older and younger patients were able to follow the ERAS guidelines. Patients aged older than 80 years were compared with those aged younger than 55 years. It was found that the compliance rates between the 2 groups were equally high (85%), and there was no difference in outcomes between these groups.[28] This also showed that reaching a high compliance rate to the ERAS Guidelines is feasible in elderly patients. Overall, most of the database studies showed no differences in outcomes between elderly and younger patients in terms of hospital stay, morbidity, or mortality. There are 2 randomized controlled trials in patients aged older than 70 years, one in open and one in laparoscopic colorectal surgery, comparing ERAS with more traditional care pathways.[29,30] Both studies showed fewer complications, a faster return of function, and a shorter hospital stay with ERAS compared with traditional care. Interestingly, in open surgery cardiac, pulmonary complications as well as urinary tract infections were less frequent in the ERAS group.

The initial results of application of ERAS in elderly patients have been confirmed in more recent literature. Moreover, more data are available on compliance with ERAS protocols in elderly and the differences in clinical outcomes. In a retrospective study, the outcome of ERAS protocols in colorectal surgery between early elderly (65–74 years) and late elderly (aged ≥75 years) were reviewed.[31] The compliance rate was high in both groups and although the late elderly group had more comorbidities, poorer baseline characteristics, and a higher overall complication rate. However, good gastrointestinal recovery and other outcomes were comparable to early elderly patients, suggesting that ERAS protocols are safe and effective in these age groups.[31,32] In several other studies in laparoscopic colorectal surgery, the same conclusion was made that ERAS protocols in elderly patients are beneficial and safe.

Recent literature also suggests that implementation of ERAS protocol in liver resection, orthopedic surgery, lung surgery, and spine surgery in elderly results in major improvements in perioperative outcomes, reduction in complications, readmissions, length of stay, and improved patient-reported outcomes and functional recovery compared with non-ERAS care.[33–36]

SUMMARY AND THOUGHTS FOR THE FUTURE

Overall, available literature shows that ERAS protocols are safe to use in older, frail, and high-risk patients, and the data available suggest that ERAS results in faster recovery, and fewer complications also in this age group. Although the overall level of scientific evidence remains sparse and, for the most part, low for this specific group of patients, large case series reflecting real-life surgical practice repeatedly report benefits from the evidence-based, low-stress impact surgical care that ERAS brings. It is very unlikely that large, randomized trials will ever be conducted to test ERAS versus traditional care. However, we are still missing knowledge about the efficacy of single ERAS elements for many types of surgery. Such studies remain a challenge for the future to help tailor ERAS for the different types of operations.

CLINICS CARE POINTS

- ERAS guidelines are especially well suited for older patients by minimizing stress
- Preadmission ERAS elements are important for this patient group to identify risks and special needs
- Malnutrition, frailty and comorbidities, are more common in older patients and often needs treatment
- Many elderly, especially frail patients, benefit from prehabilitation as part of ERAS

DISCLOSURES

O. Ljungqvist is the cofounder and past chairperson of the ERAS Society, he is the founder and shareholder of Encare AB (SE), serves as an advisor to Nutricia (NL), has received speaking honoraria from Nutricia (NL), Fresenius-Kabi (DE), BBraun (DE), Pharmacosmos (DK), and Medtronic (IT). H.D. de Boer is Chairman of the ERAS Society, he serves in the global advisory board of Merck & Co, Inc, the scientific advisory board of Senzime, the global advisory board of NMD Pharma, and he receives research grants from Merck & Co, Inc, and The Medicines Company, United States.

REFERENCES

1. Ljungqvist O, Scott M, Fearon KC. Enhanced recovery after surgery: a review. JAMA Surg 2017;152(3):292–8.
2. Bardram L, Funch-Jensen P, Jensen P, et al. Recovery after laparoscopic colonic surgery with epidural analgesia, and early oral nutrition and mobilisation. Lancet 1995;345(8952):763–4.
3. Kehlet H. Multimodal approach to control postoperative pathophysiology and rehabilitation. Br J Anaesth 1997;78(5):606–17.
4. Fearon KC, Ljungqvist O, Von Meyenfeldt M, et al. Enhanced recovery after surgery: a consensus review of clinical care for patients undergoing colonic resection. Clin Nutr 2005;24(3):466–77.

5. Gustafsson UO, Hausel J, Thorell A, et al, Enhanced Recovery After Surgery Study Group. Adherence to the enhanced recovery after surgery protocol and outcomes after colorectal cancer surgery. Arch Surg 2011;146(5):571–7.

6. Nelson G, Kiyang LN, Crumley ET, et al. Implementation of Enhanced Recovery After Surgery (ERAS) Across a Provincial Healthcare System: The ERAS Alberta Colorectal Surgery Experience. World J Surg 2016;40(5):1092–103.

7. Ripollés-Melchor J, Ramírez-Rodríguez JM, Casans-Francés R, et al. POWER Study Investigators Group for the Spanish Perioperative Audit and Research Network (REDGERM). Association between use of enhanced recovery after surgery protocol and postoperative complications in colorectal surgery: the post-operative outcomes within enhanced recovery after surgery protocol (POWER) study. JAMA Surg 2019;154(8):725–36 [Erratum in: JAMA Surg. 2022 May 1;157(5):460. PMID: 31066889; PMCID: PMC6506896].

8. Gustafsson UO, Oppelstrup H, Thorell A, et al. Adherence to the ERAS protocol is Associated with 5-year survival after colorectal cancer surgery: a retrospective cohort study. World J Surg 2016;40(7):1741–7.

9. Pisarska M, Torbicz G, Gajewska N, et al. Compliance with the ERAS Protocol and 3-Year Survival After Laparoscopic Surgery for Non-metastatic Colorectal Cancer. World J Surg 2019;43(10):2552–60.

10. Pang Q, Duan L, Jiang Y, et al. Oncologic and long-term outcomes of enhanced recovery after surgery in cancer surgeries - a systematic review. World J Surg Oncol 2021;19(1):191.

11. Varadhan KK, Neal KR, Dejong CH, et al. The enhanced recovery after surgery (ERAS) pathway for patients undergoing major elective open colorectal surgery: a meta-analysis of randomized controlled trials. Clin Nutr 2010;29(4):434–40.

12. Gillissen F, Hoff C, Maessen JM, et al. Structured synchronous implementation of an enhanced recovery program in elective colonic surgery in 33 hospitals in The Netherlands. World J Surg 2013;37(5):1082–93.

13. Ljungqvist O, Jonathan E. Rhoads lecture 2011: Insulin resistance and enhanced recovery after surgery. JPEN J Parenter Enteral Nutr 2012;36(4):389–98.

14. McIsaac DI, MacDonald DB, Aucoin SD. Frailty for perioperative clinicians: a narrative review. Anesth Analg 2020;130(6):1450–60.

15. Smilowitz NR, Berger JS. Perioperative cardiovascular risk assessment and management for noncardiac surgery: a review. JAMA 2020;324(3):279–90.

16. Cheisson G, Jacqueminet S, Cosson E, et al. working party approved by the French Society of Anaesthesia and Intensive Care Medicine (SFAR), the French Society for the study of Diabetes (SFD). Perioperative management of adult diabetic patients. Preoperative period. Anaesth Crit Care Pain Med 2018;37(Suppl 1):S9–19.

17. Ljungqvist O, de Boer HD, Balfour A, et al. Opportunities and Challenges for the Next Phase of Enhanced Recovery After Surgery: A Review. JAMA Surg 2021; 156(8):775–84 [Erratum in: JAMA Surg. 2021 Aug 1;156(8):800. PMID: 33881466].

18. Brindle M, Nelson G, Lobo DN, et al. Recommendations from the ERAS® Society for standards for the development of enhanced recovery after surgery guidelines. BJS Open 2020;4(1):157–63.

19. Ljungqvist O, Thanh NX, Nelson G. ERAS-Value based surgery. J Surg Oncol 2017;116(5):608–12.

20. Thanh NX, Chuck AW, Wasylak T, et al. An economic evaluation of the Enhanced Recovery After Surgery (ERAS) multisite implementation program for colorectal surgery in Alberta. Can J Surg 2016;59(6):415–21.

21. Joliat GR, Hübner M, Roulin D, et al. Cost analysis of enhanced recovery programs in colorectal, pancreatic, and hepatic surgery: a systematic review. World J Surg 2020;44(3):647–55.

22. Roulin D, Najjar P, Demartines N. Enhanced recovery after surgery implementation: from planning to success. J Laparoendosc Adv Surg Tech 2017;27(9):876–9.

23. Delaney CP, Fazio VW, Senagore AJ, et al. 'Fast track' postoperative management protocol for patients with high co-morbidity undergoing complex abdominal and pelvic colorectal surgery. Br J Surg 2001;88(11):1533–8.

24. Bagnall NM, Malietzis G, Kennedy RH, et al. A systematic review of enhanced recovery care after colorectal surgery in elderly patients. Colorectal Dis 2014;16(12):947–56.

25. Ljungqvist O, Hubner M. Enhanced recovery after surgery-ERAS-principles, practice and feasibility in the elderly. Aging Clin Exp Res 2018;30(3):249–52.

26. Crucitti A, Mazzari A, Tomaiuolo PM, et al. Enhanced Recovery After Surgery (ERAS) is safe, feasible and effective in elderly patients undergoing laparoscopic colorectal surgery: results of a prospective single center study. Minerva Chir 2020;75(3):157–63.

27. Slieker J, Frauche P, Jurt J, et al. Enhanced recovery ERAS for elderly: a safe and beneficial pathway in colorectal surgery. Int J Colorectal Dis 2017;32(2):215–21.

28. Pędziwiatr M, Pisarska M, Wierdak M, et al. The use of the enhanced recovery after surgery (ERAS) protocol in patients undergoing laparoscopic surgery for colorectal cancer–a comparative analysis of patients aged above 80 and below 55. Pol Przegl Chir 2015;87(11):565–72.

29. Wang Q, Suo J, Jiang J, et al. Effectiveness of fast-track rehabilitation vs conventional care in laparoscopic colorectal resection for elderly patients: a randomized trial. Colorectal Dis 2012 Aug;14(8):1009–13.

30. Jia Y, Jin G, Guo S, et al. Fast-track surgery decreases the incidence of postoperative delirium and other complications in elderly patients with colorectal carcinoma. Langenbeck's Arch Surg 2014;399(1):77–84.

31. Lohsiriwat V. Outcome of enhanced recovery after surgery (ERAS) for colorectal surgery in early elderly and late elderly patients. Ann Acad Med Singap 2019 Nov;48(11):347–53.

32. Lohsiriwat V, Lertbannaphong S, Polakla B, et al. Implementation of enhanced recovery after surgery and its increasing compliance improved 5-year overall survival in resectable stage III colorectal cancer. Updates Surg 2021;73(6):2169–79.

33. Reyes MP, Pérez BS, Díaz FJL, et al. Implementation of an ERAS protocol on elderly patients in liver resection. Cir Esp 2022. https://doi.org/10.1016/j.cireng.2022.07.019. S2173-5077(22)00265-4.

34. Frassanito L, Vergari A, Nestorini R, et al. Enhanced recovery after surgery (ERAS) in hip and knee replacement surgery: description of a multidisciplinary program to improve management of the patients undergoing major orthopedic surgery. Musculoskelet Surg 2020;104(1):87–92.

35. Mazza F, Venturino M, Turello D, et al. Enhanced recovery after surgery: adherence and outcomes in elderly patients undergoing VATS lobectomy. Gen Thorac Cardiovasc Surg 2020;68(9):1003–10.

36. Dietz N, Sharma M, Adams S, et al. Enhanced recovery after surgery (ERAS) for spine surgery: a systematic review. World Neurosurg 2019;130:415–26.

Efficiency, Safety, Quality, and Empathy

Balancing Competing Perioperative Challenges in the Elderly

William K. Hart, MD[a], John C. Klick, MD, FCCP, FCCM[a],
Mitchell H. Tsai, MD, MMM, FAACD[a,b,c,*]

KEYWORDS

- Empathy • Efficiency • Geriatric • Perioperative care • Safety • Quality

KEY POINTS

- The physiology of every major organ system is altered to some degree by the normal processes of aging, and knowledge of these changes is essential to the optimal care of the elderly patient.
- Perioperative systems behave like complex adaptive systems—more like a market or an ecosystem or a community than a factory.
- Several studies have shown improved operating room (OR) efficiency when age and American Society of Anesthesiologists physical status are used to calculate turnaround times in OR scheduling.
- The priorities for the elderly patient may be markedly different from high-volume routine ambulatory care and it may be most prudent to emphasize *empathy* above all else.

INTRODUCTION

The cohort of older Americans ranging from what Tom Brokaw once called "The Greatest Generation" to today's retiring baby boomers have earned their place as a generation to be revered by those who come after.[1] Although this group accounts for a little more than 15% of the US population, it accounts for a disproportionate percentage of patients undergoing surgery—and this population is growing—current demographic estimates show that the number of people 65 years and older will double to 95 million by 2060.[2]

[a] Department of Anesthesiology, University of Vermont Larner College of Medicine, Burlington, VT, USA; [b] Department of Orthopaedics and Rehabilitation (by courtesy), University of Vermont Larner College of Medicine, Burlington, VT, USA; [c] Department of Surgery (by courtesy), University of Vermont Larner College of Medicine, Burlington, VT, USA
* Corresponding author. Department of Anesthesiology University of Vermont Medical Center, 111 Colchester Avenue, Burlington, VT.
E-mail address: mitchell.tsai@uvmhealth.org

Anesthesiology Clin 41 (2023) 657–670
https://doi.org/10.1016/j.anclin.2023.02.011   anesthesiology.theclinics.com

As these groups continue to age in variable ways, a multitude of challenges have arisen in health care regarding the safest and most effective means of providing anesthesia services to these patients. Historically, surgery in the older patient was performed for "unequivocally necessary cases," though this obviously no longer holds true.[3] Whereas much attention has recently been directed to protecting the developing infant brain under anesthesia, a similar amount of attention is now directed to *preserving* the functioning mind and body that developed over 65 or more years.

Many of these elderly patients may be exquisitely sensitive to the effects of anesthesia and surgery and may experience cognitive and physical decline before, during, or after hospital admission. Aging compromises the function and reserve of every organ system. It produces a pro-inflammatory state and alters the pharmacokinetics and pharmacodynamics of anesthetics and other medications leading to increased risk of morbidity and mortality in the perioperative area. In this review article, the authors briefly examine the physiologic processes underlying aging. The authors then review their clinical implications through the lenses of operational efficiency, safety, and empathy.

THE PHYSIOLOGIC CHANGES OF AGING

The process of aging has substantial implications for any patient facing an anesthetic and for the anesthesiologist providing it. The physiology of every major organ system is altered to some degree by the normal processes of aging, and knowledge of these changes is essential to the optimal care of the elderly patient.

Neurologic

Widespread structural changes occur in the brain with normal aging. Atrophy is universal but most prominent in the prefrontal cortex and hippocampus and areas responsible for complex thought processes and memory. There is a reduction in synaptic density, neuronal size, and synaptic branching. With aging, there is also a reduction in neurogenesis, an imbalance of neurotransmitters, degradation of the microcirculation and glymphatic system, and dysfunction of the blood–brain barrier. The net result is that older patients' brains are less resilient to the inflammatory effects of surgical stress.[3]

The aging nervous system results in an increased incidence of perioperative neurocognitive disorders. There is ample evidence of a spectrum of cognitive declines in elderly persons occurring after surgery. Now formally classified as postoperative neurocognitive disorder (PND) it includes clinical and research definitions including postoperative disorder (POD), delayed neurocognitive recovery, neurocognitive disorder, and postoperative neurocognitive dysfunction (POCD).[4] Each of these declines in cognitive health after surgery represents a challenge to the anesthesiologist's attempts to first, do no harm. POD alone occurs in up to 65% of elderly patients[4] and in some patients is associated with permanent cognitive decline, increased morbidity and mortality, and phenomenally increases medical costs.[5,6]

Respiratory

The compliance of the lung and chest wall both decrease with age. Total lung capacity, forced vital capacity (VC), forced expiratory volume in 1 second, and VC all decrease with advancing age. Residual volume and functional residual capacity generally remain unchanged. These physiologic changes are due to the increased collapsibility of alveoli from a reduction in elastic support of the airways. By age 65, the closing capacity of the lungs starts to encroach on normal tidal volume during normal breathing.

The result is a mismatch of ventilation and perfusion and a drop in arterial oxygen tension. The loss of elastic tissue around the oropharynx leaves the elderly prone to collapse of the upper airway.[7]

Cardiovascular

Elasticity of arterial vessels decreases with age, resulting in an increase in systemic vascular resistance and hypertension. This may lead to left ventricular hypertrophy and strain. Cardiac output falls by about 3% per decade due to reductions in stroke volume and ventricular contractility. This results in a slower circulation time for intravenous anesthetics to reach the brain. Reductions in cardiac conducting cells increase the incidence of heart block, ectopy, and arrhythmias, such as atrial fibrillation. With aging, there is a downregulation of beta-adrenergic receptors in the myocardium, leading to reductions in response to beta-adrenergic catecholamine drugs. Reduced compliance of the arteries may result in a reduction in response to vasoconstrictors. Changes in the carotid baroreceptor response mean that the heart rate may not always appropriately respond to changes in blood pressure. This may result in a higher chance of hypotension from intravenous and inhalational anesthetic agents. Conversely, spinal anesthesia is often well tolerated as sympathetic blockade does not have the same degree of effect on nonelastic blood vessels.[7]

Renal Physiology

Normal aging results in a progressive loss of renal cortical glomeruli and a decrease in glomerular filtration rate. Reduced cardiac output and atherosclerotic vascular disease lead to a further decline in renal function. Prostatic hypertrophy in men can lead to obstructive nephropathy, and dehydration is common in the elderly patients during periods of illness. The reduction in muscle mass with aging may result in a deceptively normal creatinine. Creatinine clearance gives a better indication of renal function as opposed to isolated creatinine levels. Furthermore, compromised renal function leads to a reduction in drug clearance and a higher rate of electrolyte imbalance.[7]

Metabolic Disturbances

Individual basal metabolic rate falls by 1% per year after the age 30 years. This reduction in metabolic activity results in impaired thermoregulatory control and may increase the rate of perioperative hypothermia, which can lead to higher rates of infection. Shivering increases oxygen consumption, stressing organ systems. Non-insulin-dependent diabetes mellitus is present in over 25% of patients over the age of 85 years. Diabetes impairs renal and cardiac function and results in neuropathy, retinopathy, and nephropathy. Elderly patients also have a higher incidence of thyroid disorders, osteoporosis, and nutritional deficiencies.[7]

The physiologic changes of aging can also translate directly into an impact on operating room (OR) efficiency and safety.

EFFICIENCY IN THE ELDERLY

Previously, Mahajan and colleagues[8] noted that perioperative systems behave like complex adaptive systems—"more like a market or an ecosystem or a community than a factory." Today, much of the current literature related to OR management is based on the assumption that ORs resemble manufacturing plants, whereby lean manufacturing and Six Sigma approaches are used to reduce variability in clinical processes and minimize inefficiencies to create value.[9] With this highly analytical or reductionist approach, the complex parts are reduced to smaller components. This decomposition usually leads to a loss of information, especially when it comes to downstream consequences, both financial and operational.[9] These factory-style efficiencies, while essential for some patient care, may be difficult or impossible to apply in many situations to the elderly population.[10]

Over 40 years ago, Evers emphasized the importance of multidisciplinary teams when it comes to the care of the older patient.[11] In the perioperative period, these stakeholders, which may include nurses, anesthesia providers, technicians, surgeons, and hospital management, each may have different perspectives on efficiency. From a *manufacturing* perspective, efficiency focuses on using the minimal amount of resources necessary to get a task done. Alternatively, most *perioperative* discussions focus on access to care, throughput, and productivity (eg, treating the most patients possible).[9] *Scientific* management approaches use time and motion studies to find the best method for any particular task. Taylor is the founder of the modern day time-driven, activity-based costing (TDABC), whereby measuring the time it takes to perform a task and multiplying this duration by the unit cost per minute provides OR managers a tool to elucidate their operating costs.[12] Embedded in this TDABC exercise is the ongoing argument whether bottoms up or top-down based costing systems are superior and if the decision to define specific expenses as direct or indirect costs merely complicates any analysis.[13] Regarding OR management, there is underused and overused time, reflecting both fixed and variable costs.

It is now increasingly understood that the pillars of patient safety, quality, empathy, and communication in aging persons can present challenges to the production pressure and efficiency measures that govern anesthetic delivery. How do we make operational decisions when the primary stakeholder is the elderly patient? Previously, Dexter created a rational list of ordered priorities: (1) patient safety, (2) open access, (3) reduce overused time, (4) reduce underused time, and (5) surgeon satisfaction. These priorities are both tactical and operational.[14] Alternatively and perhaps more relevant to the elderly population, Hyson commented that clinical care, when viewed through OR management decisions, might look different when one applies an ethical framework.[15] It is important to remember that maintaining the production of surgery is always a priority in OR management as production is the equivalent of treating patients in need.

Anesthesiologists are tasked daily with balancing competing priorities, such as safety, quality, and efficiency to develop a rational approach to care. Yet, the priorities for the elderly patient may be markedly different from high-volume routine ambulatory care. Therefore, it may be most prudent to emphasize *empathy* above all else. This would mean that the time and flexibility required to effectively optimize comorbidities, assess cognition, and pre-habilitate and to deliver anesthetic care in a manner that truly delivers value to the elderly patients and their families requires efficiency to take a frequent back seat. This needs to be achieved while not diminishing the value of safety and quality care. In fact, several studies have shown improved OR efficiency when age and American Society of Anesthesiologists (ASA) physical status are used to calculate turnaround times in OR scheduling[16,17] with improved efficiency resulting from *increased* allocation of time to complete certain aspects of elderly anesthesia care including preoperative assessment, regional anesthetics (eg, spinal morphine), and invasive line placement (eg, arterial catheters).

In *The Theory of Constraints*, Goldratt points out that optimizing systems requires an acceptance of a bottleneck constraint.[18] For elderly patients, the bottleneck constraint may be consistently variable and unpredictable in a myriad of clinical scenarios, for example, arthritis of the spine during the placement of epidural catheters; peripheral vascular disease in arterial catheter placement; and a variety of nuanced preoperative conversations that may require more time due to presbycusis or cognitive decline. Further, complex goals of care discussions or merely a pleasant unhurried approach necessitates a willingness to abandon health care's production pressures. The anesthetic considerations of the elderly patient certainly require anesthesiologists to redefine the period of time for which they are responsible or simply acknowledge a larger investment of time. A simple consideration of the five questions proposed in Gawande's "*Being Mortal*: Medicine and What Matters in the End" can reveal tremendous information and insight in to the mindset of any patient facing serious illness.[19]

SAFETY AND QUALITY: DESIGNING SAFETY II SYSTEMS

In 2018, the American Society of Anesthesiology's Perioperative Brain Health Initiative Summary Report was published.[20] It detailed a variety of assessment tools, definitions, and recommendations for perioperative management of elderly patients. This valuable document along with the 2015 American Society of Geriatrics best practice statement and the 2018 Recommendations from the Fifth International Perioperative Neurotoxicity Working Group outline the challenges faced by those providing anesthesia and those receiving anesthesia.[21,22] Currently, the aging process in relation to anesthesia and surgery remains only modestly understood, and only a limited number of specific, data-driven recommendations for patient safety exist, whereas adherence to national recommendations is often low.[23] Many advances are currently underway to improve patient safety of vulnerable elderly patients undergoing anesthesia and surgery. Understanding the phases of anesthesia care and where to target structured improvements will be key to improving patient outcomes in elderly patients.

Preoperative

Evidence exists that early identification of preoperative cognitive decline through screening tools may be essential to targeting improvements in clinical outcomes.[24,25] These data-driven metrics can identify patients with underlying or early dementia and estimate risk of postoperative cognitive dysfunction. The preoperative anesthesia clinic is an optimal venue to explore and discuss anesthetic risks with these high-risk patients.[26] The increased incidence of common disease states can have a dramatic impact on the management of these patients and every effort should be made to optimize patients' medical conditions before undergoing anesthesia and surgery.

Frailty, a state of diminished physiologic reserve and vulnerability to stressors,[27] in particular is closely associated with poor surgical outcomes in the elderly.[28,29] It is important to appreciate that the measurement of frailty improves the accuracy of classic predictive classification schemes such as the ASA classifications and the Lee criteria.[30,31] Hall and colleagues[32] demonstrated an absolute reduction in 180-day mortality of 19% following a frailty screening initiative. The current evidence suggests that the Clinical Frailty Scale[33] may be most feasible and accurate for predicting frailty.[34]

Targeted preoperative testing should be based on the patient's comorbidities and surgical risk.[35] Few tests currently do more than increase the cost of care but may be indicated if they potentially change management. The American College of Surgeons National Surgical Quality Improvement Program (NSQIP) surgical risk calculator screening can be used to estimate surgical risk. Surgical risk greater than or equal to 1% (elevated risk) can signal the need for stress testing if functional capacity is poor (<4 metabolic equivalents).[36] Current American College of Cardiology/American Heart Association (ACC/AHA) guidelines recommend electrocardiogram (ECG), echocardiographic evaluation of left ventricular function, and exercise stress testing for patients with known cardiac disease, changes (or unknown) in functional status, new-onset shortness of breath, or elevated risk procedures.[36]

The assessment of pulmonary disease, including the presence of obstructive sleep apnea (OSA) in the elderly, can be accomplished via a variety of tests including the commonly used STOP-BANG criteria. The presence of OSA and age greater than 45 years are stand-alone risk factors for difficulty with airway management.[37] The Assess Respiratory Risk in Surgical Patients in Catalonia group developed a scoring system that can identify elevated risk for a variety of postoperative pulmonary complications. These complications occur in around 5% of surgical patients, but age over 51 years (and particularly over 80 years) as well as low preoperative SpO_2, recent respiratory tract infections, and preoperative anemia—-all things common in elderly populations accounted for the majority of risk.[38]

Functional status and malnutrition should be evaluated as well.[39] The Mini Nutritional Assessment identifies patients at severe nutritional risk.[40] Anemia, poor nutritional status, low iron, folate, and B_{12} are associated with increased perioperative complications.[41] The American Society for Enhanced Recovery and Perioperative Quality Initiative released a consensus statement in 2018 targeting several strategies for optimizing preoperative nutrition. The recommendations include screening for nutritional status and malnutrition using the perioperative nutrition screen, nutrition consults as necessary, oral, or enteral nutritional supplements emphasizing increased protein intake and the use of oral rehydration carbohydrate drinks early on the day of surgery.[42]

The Fifth International Perioperative Neurotoxicity Working Group issued the following consensus statement: All patients over age 65 years should be informed of the risks of PND including confusion, inattention, and memory problems. An evaluation of the baseline cognitive function of the individual patient is essential before any anesthetic, as general anesthesia may potentially lead to impaired postoperative cognitive function.[3] A Mini-Cog or simple assessment of orientation to name, location, and date should be performed as part of the initial assessment. In summary, the preoperative assessment of the older patient should identify patients at high risk for nutritional deficiencies, functional difficulties, and pre-habilitation efforts.[43]

Lastly, the preoperative period is also an opportune time to engage in shared decision-making. Elderly patients may be confronted with multiple reasonable options for care, and a strong physician–patient relationship can help to guide decision-making. Here, physicians may serve as experts in medical evidence and patients as experts in what matters to them. As defined by the state of Washington, shared decision-making is a process between a physician and patient where options for care are discussed in a manner that emphasizes the patient's individual preferences and values.[44] The process involves taking time to listen and understand the elderly patient's perspective and arrive at a decision for care that may include aggressive treatment but also limitations of treatment including palliative care.

Intraoperative

The normal aging process has enormous implications for the pharmacology of anesthetic drugs. Reduced cardiac output prolongs the onset time of intravenous anesthetics. The volume of distribution of drugs is reduced secondary to the reduction in total body water and increased adipose tissue. The reduction of plasma proteins results in a decreased protein binding and an increase in free drug availability. There is a decrease in the minimum alveolar concentration (MAC) of inhalational anesthetics by about 6% per decade, and elderly patients have an increased sensitivity to the central nervous system (CNS) depressant effects of anesthetic drugs.[3]

A longer period of preoxygenation is required in elderly patients before induction of general anesthesia due to decreased lung volumes, increased closing capacity, increased ventilation-perfusion mismatch, and impairment in O_2 uptake.[45] Osteoarthritis is also extremely common in the elderly population, and deformation of bones and joints may complicate the use of regional anesthetic techniques and prolong the time required to place them. Osteoporosis and age-related changes in skin collagen raise the risks of perioperative iatrogenic injury, skin breakdown, and pressure injuries.[3] Preoperative, intraoperative, and postoperative use of forced air warming blankets for maintenance of normothermia is strongly recommended.[22] Last, tight glucose control has proved more problematic than originally thought and may also lead to increased postoperative delirium.[46]

Electroencephalogram (EEG)-guided general anesthesia remains controversial, but evidence now shows that when MAC is reduced effectively by processed EEG systems, delirium rates in elderly patients can be reduced.[47] Reducing burst suppression during induction of anesthesia alone is associated with the reduced rates of POD.[48,49] The Successful Aging After Geriatric Surgery trial showed that 24% of patients developed POCD.[50] Here, POCD is associated with a significant increase in the hospital length of stay, readmission within 30 days, and a discharge to another institution.

Anesthesia and surgery are contributing to POD or cognitive dysfunction. Simply avoiding medications on the Beers Criteria list can be an easy and safe approach to anesthetic management.[51] Berger and colleagues have argued that avoiding anesthetic overdoses and closely monitoring the age-adjusted MAC fraction is necessary given the narrow therapeutic indices of inhalational agents.

Several studies have now shown no difference between general anesthesia and spinal anesthesia regarding functional outcomes and incidence of delirium.[52,53] Declines after surgery seem to be related to the surgery itself or functional declines leading up to hospitalization. Encouragingly, Whitaker and colleagues have demonstrated that the EEG patterns in pediatric patients receiving a spinal anesthetic closely resemble sleep. It is possible that the changes in sleep patterns in the aging patient may play a contributing factor to cognitive dysfunction.

Postoperative Considerations

Postoperatively, pulmonary complications are far more frequent in the elderly. Minimally invasive surgical techniques and regional anesthetic techniques may help to minimize postoperative pulmonary complications.[22] If neuromuscular blocking agents are required during the anesthetic, use should be limited to short or intermediate acting agents in any patient for whom extubation is planned. Vecuronium and rocuronium have both been shown to have prolonged durations of action in the elderly. Monitoring the depth of neuromuscular blockade becomes critically important in this patient population.[22]

Inadequate pain control postoperatively may contribute to a higher incidence of postoperative cognitive dysfunction (POCD). The judicious use of regional anesthetics and non-opioid pain relievers may help. Morphine and its derivatives remain the gold standard for acute postoperative pain management but are associated with POCD, delirium, and respiratory depression in the elderly. Non-opioid pain management strategies including dexmedetomidine, regional techniques, acetaminophen, nonsteroidal anti-inflammatory drugs, lidocaine, and ketamine are preferred. Gabapentinoids and muscle relaxants should be avoided. These medications are general CNS depressants and are risky in elderly patients who are already at a high risk for CNS depression and polypharmacy. Robust data on their efficacy in pain management are limited and the American Geriatrics Society has noted that both vecuronium and rocuronium have been shown should be avoided or used in reduced doses.[51,54] Intraoperative hypotension and hypoxia may also contribute to POCD, along with certain medications such as ketamine, benzodiazepines, and anticholinergics. The avoidance of hypoxia and hypercarbia in the postoperative setting may also help to mitigate POCD.[22]

Although more studies are necessary to determine the cost-effectiveness of various strategies to assess short- and long-term cognitive outcomes, POCD only represents the tip of the iceberg of both the burden and opportunities as it pertains to anesthesia care for this patient population. Much can be ascertained from the wide spectrum of cognitive function of older patients. By identifying the complex interplay of factors, from sleep hygiene to neuroprotection throughout the entire spectrum of perioperative care, anesthesiology as a specialty might further refine our understanding of consciousness and unconsciousness. Further, anesthesiologists might lay the groundwork to further refine anesthetic care for all patients by elucidating the factors that contribute to resilience in the older patients.

Rothenberg and colleagues[55] demonstrated that frailty is a risk factor for unplanned readmissions after elective outpatient surgery and that presence of frailty doubled the risk. Frail patients have long been shown to be more likely to be readmitted following inpatient orthopedic, general, or vascular surgery.[56–58] The implications are clear. The decision for ambulatory versus inpatient surgery needs to be decided on a case-by-case basis. Against the backdrop of decreasing reimbursements, a workforce shortage, and high occupancy rates, anesthesia providers need to convince hospital administrators that operational efficiency may need to take a back seat when it comes to the care of the elderly patient.

EMPATHY

Compassion is not a relationship between the healer and the wounded. It is a relationship between equals.

—Pema Chodron

In 1988, the Arnold P. Gold Foundation was established to promote humanism in medical school education. Empathy in the clinical setting has become a significant point of interest in medical and resident education in recent years and is deeply tied to patient-centered care. The Institute of Medicine, among others, emphasize patient-centeredness as a core attribute of a high-quality health care system.[59] Admissions committees at many US medical schools now include an evaluation of the applicant's ability to emphasize with patients in challenging simulated situations.[60,61] The value of empathy in patient care is increasingly well understood through a growing body of literature, facilitating a better definition of the term and allowed education programs in these arenas to be quantified.[62]

In *Atlas of the Heart*, Brené Brown defines compassion as "the daily practice of recognizing and accepting our shared humanity...so that we take action in the face of suffering." She points out that empathy is a skill set, one of the most engaging tools of compassion.[63] Empathy has been defined as "a predominantly cognitive (rather than an affective or emotional) attribute that involves an understanding (rather than feeling) of pain and suffering of the patient, combined with a capacity to communicate this understanding, and an intention to help."[64] Empathy is emphasized in medicine for its intention to favor cognition and understanding over emotional connections to patient which can quickly confound delivery of care. Central to empathy is the assumption that face-to-face interactions with the patient are paramount to understanding the patient's unique condition. Yet, as electronic medical records (EMR) develop and become an ever-increasing presence in the daily practice of medicine it has become common for patients to devolve into digital EMR avatars of themselves. Although this efficient extraction of medical information may be useful much of the time, the unique needs of aging patients are easy to overlook.[10]

As the American population ages and baby boomers continue to retire, the need for face-to-face communication in medicine is growing as time at the bedside and empathy are on the decline.[65] The gap in bedside empathy is being addressed with simulation[66] and curriculum development.[62] A robust humanism curriculum for anesthesiology residents was shown to increase empathy, professionalism, and overall patient satisfaction while also demonstrating reductions in anxiety and pain.[62] These qualities have been associated with reduced perioperative anxiety. Studies elsewhere have confirmed the benefits of empathy in reducing patient anxiety.[67,68] Acknowledgement, empathy, and early support were associated with lower long-term psychological complications in the UK's 5th National Audit Project report.[69] Last, simply engaging with patients will remain an essence of medicine. As Francis Peabody noted in 1927 "the care of the patient is in caring for the patient... to engage deeply with patients... see the sorrows of severe illness, the hardships and resources of the family, and the circumstances of our patients' lives."[70]

THE IMMUTABLE PROGRESSION OF DEMOGRAPHY

You get old and you realize there are no answers, just stories.
—Garrison Keillor

With the Great Resignation underway, we believe that anesthesiologists should take a step back when it comes to the anesthetic care of the elderly patient. There is a current physician shortage, and as a specialty, anesthesiologists represent a very small segment of the active practicing physicians in the country and possibly the world. Currently, there are 6,000,000 surgeries waiting to be performed in the National Health Service (England) and 150,000,000 around the world.[71,72] For the United States, anesthesiology departments and health care systems are dealing with a shortage of anesthesiologists not only as a result of demographics but also because of short-sighted health care policy proposals in the 1990s leading to a dearth of medical students seeking training as an anesthesiologist.

As the leaders of patient safety, anesthesiologists should recognize that our past successes should build the foundation for future avenues to improve patient care.[73] Further, the recent pandemic has shown that operational efficiency and maximizing profits is meaningless against the backdrop of a broken health care system. Gawande exhorts physicians to recognize not only their patient's mortality but also their own.[19] We hope that readers of this review article will recognize that empathy and safety trumps efficiency, always. As anesthesiologists, we occupy a twilight zone between sheer panic and a patient's potential future. And perhaps, one day, we, ourselves, would like to be approached by an anesthesia provider, less concerned about operational efficiency, and more empathetic to the idea that there are always many unknown unknowns. As Giam recently remarked "most patients will never know the amount of scientific and professional education and personal sacrifice it takes to become an anesthesiologist, but they *will* remember the art and the humanity of a caring physician."

SUMMARY

Any survival benefit associated with the surgical care of the elderly population will most likely require multidisciplinary, collaborative efforts, from the preoperative decision-making process, fine-tuning the intraoperative workflows, and building the postoperative monitoring necessary to minimize the impact of surgery and anesthesia. There is much opportunity to improve the quality of anesthesiology's contribution to our patients' experiences and outcomes. Anesthesiologists can best advocate for our patients when we function as a part of their perioperative clinical team and as leaders of patient safety,.Taking the opportunity to continually refine our clinical practice for the elderly patient may create new avenues to demonstrate our value as a specialty.

CLINICS CARE POINTS

- Elderly patients may require an increased allocation of block time for unhurried preoperative admission and assessment, intraoperative and postoperative management. Better block time allocation for elderly patients in surgery can reduce operating room inefficiency.

- Optimizing patients preoperatively may include aspects of nutrition, cognitive, and physical pre-habilitation and assessment for cognitive decline. These early investments in the preoperative clinic may lead to reduced delirium and improved safety and outcomes.

- An aspect of slowing down the perioperative juggernaut may be necessary to improve care in elderly patients by taking extra time for empathy and value-based discussions that may include goals of care, shared decision-making, and discussions regarding reasonable expectations and outcomes.

CONTRIBUTION

The author helped create the article and provided critical edits.

ATTESTATION

All the authors approve the article as submitted.

CONFLICTS OF INTEREST

None.

REFERENCES

1. Brokaw T. The greatest generation. New York: Random House; 1998.
2. Centers for Disease Control and Prevention. 65 and Older Population Grows Rapidly as Baby Boomers Age; Available at: https://www.census.gov/newsroom/press-releases/2020/65-older-population-grows.html, 2020. Accessed August 2, 2022.
3. Vacas S., Canales C., Deiner S.G., et al., Perioperative Brain Health in the Older Adult: A Patient Safety Imperative, Anesth Analg, 135 (2), 2022, 316–328.
4. Rudolph JL, Marcantonio ER. Review articles: postoperative delirium: acute change with long-term implications. Anesth Analg 2011;112(5):1202–11.
5. Leslie DL, Inouye SK. The importance of delirium: economic and societal costs. J Am Geriatr Soc 2011;59(Suppl 2):S241–3.
6. Leslie D.L., Marcantonio E.R., Zhang Y., et al., One-year health care costs associated with delirium in the elderly population, Arch Intern Med, 168 (1), 2008, 27–32.

7. Anatomy and physiology of Ageing. World Anaesthesia Tutorial of the Week. 2006. In AnaesthesiaUK, Fellowship of the Royal College of Anaesthetists. https://www.anaesthesiauk.com/article.aspx?articleid=100697.   Accessed August 22, 2022.

8. Mahajan A, Islam SD. Schwartz MJ, et al., A Hospital Is Not Just a Factory, but a Complex Adaptive System-Implications for Perioperative Care. Anesth Analg 2017;125(1):333–41.

9. Tsai M.H., Kimatian S.J., Duguay J.R., et al., Rethinking Operating Room Management: Why Clinical Directors Should Embrace Complexity, *Anesth Analg*, 131 (3), 2020, 984–988.

10. Cooper L., Lirk P., Bader A., et al., Efficiency in Elderhood, *Anesth Analg*, 135 (2), 2022, 435–437.

11. Evers HK. Multidisciplinary teams in geriatric wards: myth or reality? J Adv Nurs 1981;6(3):205–14.

12. Stewart M. *The Management Myth: Debunking Modern Business Philosophy.* New York, NY: WW Norton & Company; 2009.

13. Glenn DM, Macario A. Management of the operating room: a new practice opportunity for anesthesiologists. *Anesthesiology Clinics of North.* America 1999;17(2): 365–94.

14. Dexter F, Willemsen-Dunlap A, Lee JD. Operating room managerial decision-making on the day of surgery with and without computer recommendations and status displays. Anesth Analg 2007;105(2):419–29.

15. Hyson P, Macauley R, Sexton K, et al. Surgical Overlap: An Ethical Approach to Empirical Ambiguity. Int Anesthesiol Clin 2019;57(1):18–31.

16. Ehrenwerth J, Escobar A, Davis EA, et al. Can the attending anesthesiologist accurately predict the duration of anesthesia induction? Anesth Analg 2006; 103(4):938–40.

17. Luedi MM, Kauf P, Mulks L, et al. Implications of Patient Age and ASA Physical Status for Operating Room Management Decisions. Anesth Analg 2016;122(4): 1169–77.

18. Goldratt EM. *The Goal.* North River Press; 1984.

19. Gawande A. Being mortal : medicine and what matters in the end, First edition, New York.

20. Cole DJ, Kharasch ED. Postoperative Brain Function: Toward a Better Understanding and the American Society of Anesthesiologists Perioperative Brain Health Initiative. Anesthesiology 2018;129(5):861–3.

21. American Geriatrics Society Expert Panel on Postoperative Delirium in Older A. Postoperative delirium in older adults: best practice statement from the American Geriatrics Society. *J Am Coll Surg.* 2015;220(2):136-148 e131.

22. Berger M, Schenning KJ, Brown C, et al. Best Practices for Postoperative Brain Health: Recommendations From the Fifth International Perioperative Neurotoxicity Working Group. Anesth Analg 2018;127(6):1406–13.

23. Deiner S., Fleisher L.A., Leung J.M., et al., Adherence to recommended practices for perioperative anesthesia care for older adults among US anesthesiologists: results from the ASA Committee on Geriatric Anesthesia-Perioperative Brain Health Initiative ASA member survey. *Perioper Med (Lond).* 2020;9:6.

24. Gregory S.H., King C.R., Ben Abdallah A., et al., Abnormal preoperative cognitive screening in aged surgical patients: a retrospective cohort analysis, *Br J Anaesth*, 126 (1), 2021, 230–237.

25. Susano MJ, Grasfield RH, Friese M, et al. Brief Preoperative Screening for Frailty and Cognitive Impairment Predicts Delirium after Spine Surgery. Anesthesiology 2020;133(6):1184–91.
26. Goldenberg E, Saffary R, Schmiesing C. New Role for the Anesthesia Preoperative Clinic: Helping to Ensure That Surgery Is the Right Choice for Patients With Serious Illness. Anesth Analg 2019;129(1):311–5.
27. Adeleke I, Blitz J. Perioperative frailty: lessons learned and future directions. Curr Opin Anaesthesiol 2021;34(3):373–80.
28. Fried LP, Tangen CM, Walston J, et al. Frailty in older adults: evidence for a phenotype. J Gerontol A Biol Sci Med Sci 2001;56(3):M146–56.
29. Lin HS, Watts JN, Peel NM, et al. Frailty and post-operative outcomes in older surgical patients: a systematic review. BMC Geriatr 2016;16(1):157.
30. Makary MA, Segev DL, Pronovost PJ, et al. Frailty as a predictor of surgical outcomes in older patients. J Am Coll Surg 2010;210(6):901–8.
31. Robinson T.N., Wallace J.I., Wu D.S., et al., Accumulated frailty characteristics predict postoperative discharge institutionalization in the geriatric patient. *J Am Coll Surg.* 2011;213(1):37-42; discussion 42-34.
32. Hall DE, Arya S, Schmid KK, et al. Association of a Frailty Screening Initiative With Postoperative Survival at 30, 180, and 365 Days. JAMA Surg 2017;152(3):233–40.
33. Rockwood K, Song X, MacKnight C, et al. A global clinical measure of fitness and frailty in elderly people. CMAJ 2005;173(5):489–95.
34. Aucoin SD, Hao M, Sohi R, et al. Accuracy and Feasibility of Clinically Applied Frailty Instruments before Surgery: A Systematic Review and Meta-analysis. Anesthesiology 2020;133(1):78–95.
35. Fischer SP. Development and effectiveness of an anesthesia preoperative evaluation clinic in a teaching hospital. Anesthesiology 1996;85(1):196–206.
36. Fleisher L.A., Fleischmann K.E., Auerbach A.D., et al., 2014 ACC/AHA guideline on perioperative cardiovascular evaluation and management of patients undergoing noncardiac surgery: a report of the American College of Cardiology/American Heart Association Task Force on practice guidelines. *J Am Coll Cardiol.* 2014;64(22):e77-137.
37. Kheterpal S, Healy D, Aziz MF, et al. Incidence, predictors, and outcome of difficult mask ventilation combined with difficult laryngoscopy: a report from the multicenter perioperative outcomes group. Anesthesiology 2013;119(6):1360–9.
38. Canet J, Gallart L, Gomar C, et al. Prediction of postoperative pulmonary complications in a population-based surgical cohort. Anesthesiology 2010;113(6):1338–50.
39. Barnett SR. Preoperative Assessment of Older Adults. Anesthesiol Clin 2019;37(3):423–36.
40. Vellas B., Villars H., Abellan G., et al., Overview of the MNA–Its history and challenges. *J Nutr Health Aging.* 2006;10(6):456-463; discussion 463-455.
41. Williams DGA, Villalta E, Aronson S, et al. Development and Implementation of a Multidisciplinary Preoperative Nutrition Optimization Clinic. JPEN J Parenter Enteral Nutr 2020;44(7):1185–96.
42. Wischmeyer PE, Carli F, Evans DC, et al. American Society for Enhanced Recovery and Perioperative Quality Initiative Joint Consensus Statement on Nutrition Screening and Therapy Within a Surgical Enhanced Recovery Pathway. Anesth Analg 2018;126(6):1883–95.
43. Oresanya LB, Lyons WL, Finlayson E. Preoperative assessment of the older patient: a narrative review. JAMA 2014;311(20):2110–20.

44. Spatz ES, Krumholz HM, Moulton BW. Prime Time for Shared Decision Making. JAMA 2017;317(13):1309–10.
45. Nimmagadda U, Salem MR, Crystal GJ. Preoxygenation: Physiologic Basis, Benefits, and Potential Risks. Anesth Analg 2017;124(2):507–17.
46. Saager L, Duncan AE, Yared JP, et al. Intraoperative tight glucose control using hyperinsulinemic normoglycemia increases delirium after cardiac surgery. Anesthesiology 2015;122(6):1214–23.
47. Chan MT, Cheng BC, Lee TM, et al. BIS-guided anesthesia decreases postoperative delirium and cognitive decline. J Neurosurg Anesthesiol 2013;25(1):33–42.
48. Soehle M, Dittmann A, Ellerkmann RK, et al. Intraoperative burst suppression is associated with postoperative delirium following cardiac surgery: a prospective, observational study. BMC Anesthesiol 2015;15:61.
49. Wildes TS, Winter AC, Maybrier HR, et al. Protocol for the Electroencephalography Guidance of Anesthesia to Alleviate Geriatric Syndromes (ENGAGES) study: a pragmatic, randomised clinical trial. BMJ Open 2016;6(6):e011505.
50. Schmitt EM, Saczynski JS, Kosar CM, et al. The Successful Aging after Elective Surgery (SAGES) Study: Cohort Description and Data Quality Procedures. J Am Geriatr Soc 2015;63(12):2463–71.
51. By the American Geriatrics Society Beers Criteria Update Expert P. American Geriatrics Society 2015 Updated Beers Criteria for Potentially Inappropriate Medication Use in Older Adults. J Am Geriatr Soc 2015;63(11):2227–46.
52. Neuman MD, Feng R, Carson JL, et al. Spinal Anesthesia or General Anesthesia for Hip Surgery in Older Adults. N Engl J Med 2021;385(22):2025–35.
53. Silbert BS, Evered LA, Scott DA. Incidence of postoperative cognitive dysfunction after general or spinal anaesthesia for extracorporeal shock wave lithotripsy. Br J Anaesth 2014;113(5):784–91.
54. Wilson S.H., Wilson P.R., Bridges K.H., et al., Nonopioid Analgesics for the Perioperative Geriatric Patient: A Narrative Review, Anesth Analg, 135 (2), 2022, 290–306.
55. Rothenberg KA, Stern JR, George EL, et al. Association of Frailty and Postoperative Complications With Unplanned Readmissions After Elective Outpatient Surgery. JAMA Netw Open 2019;2(5):e194330.
56. Wahl TS, Graham LA, Hawn MT, et al. Association of the Modified Frailty Index With 30-Day Surgical Readmission. JAMA Surg 2017;152(8):749–57.
57. Robinson TN, Wu DS, Pointer L, et al. Simple frailty score predicts postoperative complications across surgical specialties. Am J Surg 2013;206(4):544–50.
58. Choe YR, Joh JY, Kim YP. Association between frailty and readmission within one year after gastrectomy in older patients with gastric cancer. J Geriatr Oncol 2017;8(3):185–9.
59. Institute of Medicine (U.S.). Committee on Quality of Health Care in America. Crossing the quality chasm : a new health system for the 21st century. Washington, D.C: National Academy Press; 2001.
60. Dore KL, Reiter HI, Kreuger S, et al. an online pre-interview screen for personal/professional characteristics: prediction of national licensure scores. Adv Health Sci Educ Theory Pract 2017;22(2):327–36.
61. Patterson F., Ashworth V., Zibarras L., et al., Evaluations of situational judgement tests to assess non-academic attributes in selection, Med Educ, 46 (9), 2012, 850–868.
62. Canales C, Strom S, Anderson CT, et al. Humanistic medicine in anaesthesiology: development and assessment of a curriculum in humanism for postgraduate anaesthesiology trainees. Br J Anaesth 2019;123(6):887–97.

63. Brown B. *Atlas of the heart : mapping meaningful connection & the language of human experience*. New York: Random House; 2021.

64. Hojat M, DeSantis J, Shannon SC, et al. The Jefferson Scale of Empathy: a nationwide study of measurement properties, underlying components, latent variable structure, and national norms in medical students. Adv Health Sci Educ Theory Pract 2018;23(5):899–920.

65. Neumann M, Edelhauser F, Tauschel D, et al. Empathy decline and its reasons: a systematic review of studies with medical students and residents. Acad Med 2011;86(8):996–1009.

66. Saiva A., Abdool P.S., Naismith L.M., et al., An Immersive Simulation to Build Empathy for Geriatric Patients with Co-Occurring Physical and Mental Illness, *Acad Psychiatry*, 44 (6), 2020, 745–750.

67. Choi SM, Lee J, Park YS, et al. Effect of Verbal Empathy and Touch on Anxiety Relief in Patients Undergoing Flexible Bronchoscopy: Can Empathy Reduce Patients, *Anxiety?* Respiration 2016;92(6):380–8.

68. van Dulmen S, van den Brink-Muinen A. Patients' preferences and experiences in handling emotions: a study on communication sequences in primary care medical visits. Patient Educ Couns 2004;55(1):149–52.

69. Pandit JJ, Andrade J, Bogod DG, et al. 5th National Audit Project (NAP5) on accidental awareness during general anaesthesia: summary of main findings and risk factors. Br J Anaesth 2014;113(4):549–59.

70. Peabody FW. The care of the patient. JAMA 2015;313(18):1868.

71. Pandit JJ, The NHS. Improvement report on operating theatres: really 'getting it right first time'? Anaesthesia 2019;74(7):839–44.

72. Model Health System. Spotlight on theatres – navigating and interpreting. model.nhs.uk. Available at: https://feedback.model.nhs.uk/knowledgebase/articles/1982208-spotlight-on-theatres Accessed September 26, 2022.

73. Sherrer DM, Franklin AD, Kimatian SJ, et al. The Icarus paradox and the future of anesthesiology. Anesth Analg 2023;136(1):185–9.

Pain Management in the Elderly: A Narrative Review

Kanishka Rajput, MD, FASA*, Jessica Ng, MD,
Nicholas Zwolinski, MD, Robert M. Chow, MD

KEYWORDS

- Pain management • Elderly • Geriatric pain • Postoperative pain
- Interventional pain

KEY POINTS

- Pain assessment and treatment remains challenging in the elderly population.
- Elderly patients underreport pain, assuming it to be a normal part of aging, and physicians undertreat pain.
- Nonpharmacologic and interventional options for management of pain, besides medications, need to be further studied in the elderly population.

INTRODUCTION

With an increase in life expectancy in the United States, octogenarians and nonagenarians are seen more frequently in clinical practice. The elderly population is projected to make up 20% of the total US population by the year 2030. The 2016 US Census Bureau estimated the number of people in the United States aged 65 years and older as 49.2 million, with greater than 50% between the ages of 65 and 74 years and 29% between the ages of 75 and 84 years.[1]

Approximately 66% of people older than 65 years report chronic pain of some type. The rate is higher for those suffering from other chronic illnesses and living in nursing homes.[2] Poorly controlled pain interferes with activities of daily living, decreases ambulation, causes mood disturbances, and increases cognitive decline. Collectively, these comorbidities could lead to other morbidities, such as deep vein thrombosis, pulmonary embolism, fractures, and poor quality of life.[3] Not only is pain underreported by the elderly, it is often assumed to be a normal part of aging.[4] In addition, pain is undertreated by physicians,[5] despite newer guidelines established for the treatment of chronic pain in the geriatric population.[6] In one study on prevalence of pain in elderly hospitalized patients, only 49% of those with pain had any type of treatment that was adequate for the pain intensity, whereas 74.5% of patients considered the therapy to be of low or no efficacy.[5]

Department of Anesthesiology, Yale University School of Medicine, 333 Cedar Street, TMP3, New Haven, CT 06510, USA
* Corresponding author.
E-mail address: kanishka.rajput@yale.edu

Anesthesiology Clin 41 (2023) 671–691
https://doi.org/10.1016/j.anclin.2023.03.003
1932-2275/23/© 2023 Elsevier Inc. All rights reserved.

Assessment and management of pain in elderly patients is often difficult given the high incidence of dementia, sensory impairment, and disability. Achieving an adequate pain management regimen for the elderly is further complicated by the presence of multiple comorbidities, increased risk of adverse drug reactions, and physician factors such as inadequate training and reluctance to prescribe opioids.

This review focuses on describing the prevalence of pain in the elderly, cause, and the optimal tools for assessment and management of pain including nonpharmacologic, pharmacologic, and interventional options.

METHODS

The authors performed a comprehensive search using Pubmed, Scopus, and Cochrane databases using the search terms "pain management" and "elderly," limiting our search to the year 2000 onward for the most recent evidence on the topic. Our initial search retrieved 4411 articles. All relevant articles pertaining to this narrative review were collated, and the best practice evidence is highlighted.

PREVALANCE

The prevalence of pain varies with age, living arrangements, and the general health status of the population. One reason for the lack of a systematic epidemiologic investigation is that pain is often considered a part of normal aging, resulting in underreporting by patients and undertreatment by physicians, even though, in the absence of disease, pain is not a normal part of aging.[7]

The incidence of pain more than doubles after age 60 years, and reported frequency of pain increases with each decade.[6] The prevalence of chronic pain increases with age up to the seventh decade[8,9] and seems to plateau after age 65 years when adjusting for other comorbidities and characteristics.[10] Pain prevalence may increase again as older adults approach the end of life.[11] Several population-based studies suggest that pain-related problems are present in 25% to 50% of community-dwelling elderly people. In the residential care setting, more than 80% of nursing home residents report chronic pain.[12] People living in long-term care facilities may also have the highest rates of undertreated pain, reported to be from 45% to 83%.[5] In addition, pain remains especially undertreated in the oldest old, African Americans and other ethnic minorities, and those with cognitive impairment.[13] Bothersome pains in elderly disproportionately affect women more than men, and 67% of community dwellers report pain of moderate or greater intensity.[14,15]

CAUSE AND PATHOGENESIS

Pain perception changes among older adults, resulting from an aging process that affects functioning at the cellular, tissue, organ system, and population levels. Moreover, there is wide interindividual variation to pain perception among older individuals.[16] The heterogeneity that exists among the physiologic, psychological, and functional capacities of older persons is clinically apparent when comparing a "healthy" octogenarian with a "frail" septuagenarian: chronologic advances in age may increase the risk of disease, but aging itself is not a disease.[17]

Pain Signaling and Aging

Changes associated with pain signaling include decreases in both molecular and cellular components that form the nociceptive pathways. In the peripheral nervous system, damaged functioning of nociceptive nerves may result from a loss of integrity or decreased concentration of neurotransmitters such as substance P and calcitonin gene–related peptide. In the central nervous system, reductions in several critical neurotransmitters such as endorphins, γ-aminobutyric acid, serotonin, norepinephrine, opioids, and acetylcholine, among others, likely result in altered pain signal transmission and neuromodulation.[18] Moreover, aging results in dysfunction of the descending modulatory pathways of the spinal dorsal columns, which normally serve as an endogenous pain inhibitory system.

Although alterations in pain perception with aging is an area of controversy, a large meta-analysis suggests that among older adults the pain threshold increases and pain tolerance decreases.[19] The threshold for pain may vary based on the type of stimulus (increased with heat, no change with electrical stimulation, decrease with mechanical pressure and ischemia), duration (increase with shorter duration), and location (increase at peripheral or visceral site).[18,20,21] Although pain may not serve as a reliable warning sign of tissue damage in some atypical clinical presentations (cardiac ischemic pain, abdominal pain) because of the increased pain threshold, this finding should not lead to the conclusion that most of the elderly population will not experience pain.[22,23] Rather, the increased pain threshold that accompanies aging may imply that more significant levels of underlying pathologic disorder may be present in older adults who endorse pain.

Common Causes of Chronic Pain in the Elderly

The most common causes of chronic pain in the elderly are listed in **Table 1**.[24]

Osteoarthritis

Osteoarthritis (OA) affects up to 50% of the elderly, and predisposing factors such as obesity are likely to increase the prevalence over the next decades. Arthritis of the knee, hip, and hand are most common conditions affecting the elderly.[25] Although various causes of OA have been studied, including joint injury and some contributing genetic factors (such as inheritance of the heterogenous allele Col2A1[26]), the strongest single identified risk factor for the development of OA is patient age.[27] Rheumatoid arthritis (RA) resulting from chronic inflammation of synovial membranes of

Table 1	
Common causes of chronic pain in elderly with associated elderly prevalence rates[24]	
Arthritis and Related Arthritides	Osteoarthritis – PR 33%–50% Rheumatoid arthritis – PR 25% (majority female) Spinal canal stenosis – PR varied, up to 47%
Neuropathic Pain Syndromes	Diabetic peripheral neuropathy – PR 40%–50% Postherpetic neuralgia (shingles) – PR up to 30% (80 yrs) Trigeminal neuralgia – PR appr. 0.2%
Malignancy Related	Cancer-related pain – PR 64% • Chemotherapy-induced peripheral neuropathy • Radiation-induced neuropathy
Vascular Causes	Peripheral vascular disease – PR 4.7% ages 60–69, 14.5% age 70+ Central poststroke pain – PR up to 50% of stroke patients
Other Causes	Myofascial pain – PR ~ 13% Fibromyalgia – 7% Postsurgical pain – PR varied

Data from Bicket MC, Mao J. Chronic pain in older adults. Anesthesiol Clin. 2015;33(3):577-590.

articular cartilage and juxta-articular bone is less prevalent in the elderly than OA. The reported prevalence rate of OA is 26% in the elderly, and nearly 75% of those afflicted are women.[28] Patients often present with bilateral painful swelling of joints of the hands and feet, primarily in the wrists, metacarpophalangeal, and proximal interphalangeal joints.[29]

Spinal canal stenosis
Spinal canal stenosis presenting as recurrent or chronic pain with or without neurogenic claudication most commonly affects the lumbar and cervical regions. It represents the most frequent indication for surgical intervention in patients 65 years and older.[30] Although radiological evidence of acquired spinal canal stenosis may present much earlier, most cases of spinal canal stenosis only become symptomatic after the sixth decade of life.[31] Some degree of radiological evidence of stenosis exists in up to 80% of individuals older than 70 years; however, this does not necessarily correlate directly with symptoms; one-fifth of nonsymptomatic patients aged 60 years and older will demonstrate at least some stenosis on MRI.[32] Lumbar stenosis incidence is known to be 4 times higher than cervical stenosis, and cervical and lumbar stenosis coexist in 5% of patients.

Diabetic neuropathy
The prevalence of diabetic neuropathy (DN) increases with age. Duration of diabetes less than 5 years is associated with prevalence of 20.8% of DN, whereas duration of diabetes greater than 10 years is associated with prevalence of 36.8% of DN. By the time a diabetic patient reaches the age of 65 years and is deemed elderly, their overall risk of neuropathic pain is 61.5%, which is an 8.6% higher prevalence of pain compared with the general population, when matched for the age group.[10] The prevalence of pain is 10% to 20% in patients with diabetes alone and from 40% to 50% in those with diabetic neuropathy.[33]

Postherpetic neuralgia
Postherpetic neuralgia (PHN) is another common neuropathic pain syndrome afflicting the elderly. After infection by varicella zoster virus and subsequent dormancy of the virus in the dorsal root ganglion, incidence of reactivation increases with age; this is thought to be due to coincident decline in cell-mediated immunity with aging. Of patients with varicella zoster reactivation (shingles), 10% will progress to develop PHN, and risk increases to 30%, once a patient reaches 80 years of age.[34]

Peripheral vascular disease
Chronic pain from peripheral vascular disease (PVD) in the elderly presents as intermittent claudication (IC).[35] This pain is experienced in the bilateral posterior calves. It is diagnosed, and its severity is assessed by performing the ankle-brachial indices. Prevalence of pain from IC is closely associated to the prevalence rate of PVD. The prevalence of PVD (and thus, pain from IC) was shown to be 4.7% for ages 60 to 69 years and 14.5% for those aged 70 years and older.[36]

Trigeminal neuralgia
Trigeminal neuralgia (TN) is a rare condition and hence the paucity of epidemiologic data. Suggested TN prevalence indicates a range of 0.03% to 0.3% in the general population, with a women to men ratio between 2:1 and 3:1.[37] Ninety percent of patients exhibit symptoms after the age of 40 years, with incidence progressing with age: 60 to 69 years demonstrate 17.5 per 100,000 annually, increasing to 25.6 per 100,000 annually after the age of 70 years. Most patients experience symptomatic attacks affecting the maxillary and mandibular trigeminal branches (V2 and V3);

however, ophthalmic branch (V1) symptoms can occur in up to 5% of patients.[38] It should be noted that interaction between chronic pain states with TN exists, namely that patients with multiple sclerosis (MS) exhibit greater incidence of TN than the general population. As many as 2% of patients with TN also have associated MS.

Poststroke pain

About 50% of poststroke patients can exhibit some form of chronic pain syndrome,[39] with as many as 70% of those affected experiencing significant enough symptoms that affects their daily lives.[40] The types of pain reported fall into categories such as musculoskeletal pain, nociceptive pain, or central poststroke pain, which includes pain secondary to spasticity, complex regional pain syndrome, or headaches. Generally, age is an independent risk factor for development of PSP, and incidence of PSP increases with the age at the time of stroke onset.[41]

Cancer-related pain

Cancer-related pain is widely studied and heterogenous in nature. One meta-analysis collated 54 studies reporting pain prevalence of 64% among patients with advanced cancer.[42] Importantly, more than one-third of these patients were subcategorized as having either moderate or severe pain, indicating substantial impact on their quality of life. These studies characterized cancer-related pain into various categories such as neuropathic, incident or breakthrough, and generalized bone pain.[43] Such studies inherently encompass treatment-related pain such as chemotherapy and radiation therapy–induced pain. The category of cancer-related pain is likely to expand as treatment of cancers advance in the elderly and prolong life.[44]

Miscellaneous chronic pain causes in the elderly

The remainder of other chronic pain causes include myofascial pain (prevalence of 13.8%),[45] fibromyalgia (prevalence of 2.1% to 7.1%),[35] and chronic postsurgical pain. Postsurgical pain can progress past the acute phase and develop into chronic pain when duration exceeds 2 months from the time of surgery, generally seen after amputations, coronary bypass surgeries.[46] Although controversial, younger age has been identified as a consistent risk factor for the development of chronic postsurgical pain when compared with elderly groups.[47,48]

PAIN ASSESSMENT TOOLS

Assessment of pain in the elderly should begin with a comprehensive medical history and physical examination (**Table 2**).[49] Elderly patients likely have more than one cause contributing to their chronic pain. Frequently, treatment of one causative factor will not necessarily address all aspects of a patient's experience of chronic pain. Therefore, treatment of elderly chronic pain requires addressing multiple sources of their pain through comprehensive evaluation and treatment.[50] In addition, the diminished physiologic reserve and loss of pain as a warning sign in some older adults may increase the likelihood of atypical presentations of chronic pain.[51]

The best indicator of pain in the elderly remains a person's self-reported pain level, and several assessment tools for pain intensity have been validated in this population (**Table 3**).[52] Mild to moderate cognitive impairment, common to conditions such as dementia, does not impair the appropriate use of these tools in most situations.[53] The most common scales used in practice are the numerical rating scales (NRS), the visual analogue scales (VAS), and the verbal descriptor scales (VDS). NRS describes pain by a series of numbers on an 11-point scale from 0 to 10, with 0 being no pain, 10 being the worst pain possible, and the numbers in between representing

Table 2
Overview of a comprehensive pain assessment tool[49]

Domain	Components
Pain presence	At rest, with activity
Pain characteristics	Location, frequency, exacerbating and relieving factors, character, and natural history
Pain intensity	Now, on an average day, worst pain, lowest level of pain
Type of pain	Nociceptive, neuropathic, or mixed
Pain interference with activity and pain-related morbidity	Physical, psychological, spiritual, and social functioning, falls, sleep, appetite, and so forth
Cause	Osteoarthritis, osteoporosis, previous bone fractures, diabetic neuropathy, postherpetic neuralgia, myofascial pain syndromes, and so forth
Pain behaviors	Facial expressions, vocalizations, body movements, changes in interpersonal interactions and routines, and mental status changes
Pain treatment	Nonpharmacologic and pharmacologic including injections, surgical interventions, and alternative therapies
Coping style	Distraction, ignoring pain sensations, reinterpreting pain sensations, catastrophizing, praying, and hoping
Sensory	Hearing, vision, and cognition
Proxy report	Professional and family caregiver

Data from Malec M, Shega JW. Pain Management in the Elderly. Med Clin. 2015;99(2):337-350. doi:.

Table 3
Common pain behaviors in cognitively impaired older persons

Facial expressions	Frown; sad, frightened face Grimace, wrinkled forehead, closed or tightened eyes Rapid blinking
Verbalizations, vocalizations	Sighing, moaning, groaning, grunting Calling out, asking for help Noisy breathing, verbally abusive
Body movements	Rigid, tense body posture, guarding Fidgeting, increased pacing, rocking Restricted movement, gait, or mobility changes
Changes in interpersonal interactions	Aggressive, combative, resisting care Decreased social interactions Socially inappropriate, disruptive, withdrawn
Changes in activity patterns or routines	Refusing food, appetite change Sleep, rest pattern changes Sudden cessation of common routines Increased wandering
Mental status changes	Crying or tears Increased confusion Irritability or distress

Data from AGS panel on persistent pain in older persons. Society AG. Panel on Persistent Pain in Older Persons. The management of persistent pain in older adults. J Am Geriatr Soc. 2002;50(6):205-224[57] intermediate intensities.[54] VAS is a visual image that helps qualify pain states. Some studies have shown an association with VAS and unscorable responses in the elderly, so this type of scale should be used with caution.[55] On the contrary, in clinical and research settings, VAS has proved to be a useful measurement of pain because of its simplicity, reliability, and ease of use.[9] VDS describes subjective pain by using terms along a broad scale such as none, mild, moderate, strong, and worst pain possible.[56] An advantage of VDS is its simplicity of use because it is suitable for even mild to moderately impaired elderly patients. A drawback of VDS is that the terms used might have different meaning for different patients, leading to a potentially inaccurate scale. Furthermore, pain levels may vary frequently within a given day in the elderly, leading to the need for frequent assessment, to maintain desired control.

In addition, older adults with cognitive impairment may demonstrate a variety of behaviors to communicate pain, including facial expressions, verbalization, body movements, and changes in interactions with other people and their environment (**Table 4**).[57] Given the variation in pain behaviors with cognitive impairment, pain may be underappreciated and undertreated in this population.[51] Assessing pain levels or behaviors is most effectively performed during a movement-based task or when compared with a preexisting baseline state.[52] In addition, caregivers may provide ancillary information relevant to pain assessment for adults with cognitive impairment.

Outcome measures besides pain level provide important information regarding the impact of chronic pain and its treatment in all populations, but especially in older adults. Assessment of functional status including activities of daily living, mobility, sleep, appetite, weight changes, mood (including screening for anxiety, depression, and risk of suicide), and cognitive impairment (dementia or delirium) is necessary.[52] Adequate pain management is expected to result in improvements in one or more of these domains, as untreated or undertreated pain may contribute to or worsen the conditions in these domains.[58]

PAIN MANAGEMENT IN INPATIENT SETTINGS
Perioperative Pain Management

The number of elderly patients undergoing surgery in increasing. Aging affects every organ system, worsens surgical outcomes, and lends itself to a unique set of complications, including opioid sensitivity, postoperative delirium, and functional decline.[59] Thus, the elderly represents a vulnerable population with unique perioperative pain management needs. Evaluation and management of pain in the elderly patients should focus on pain history, physical examination, comprehensive education, and utilization of opioid-sparing and multimodal pain management techniques.

Factors to consider during initial evaluation include a history of chronic pain, pharmacologic, and nonpharmacologic strategies that have worked or not worked in the past and the preferences for pain control.[59] It is important to inquire about substance abuse history (eg, benzodiazepines, opioids, alcohol) and if there is a history of chronic opioid use, tolerance, or addiction. It is estimated that 6% to 9% of community-dwelling elderly use opioids, and up to 70% of nursing home elderly with chronic non-cancer pain receive regularly scheduled opioids.[60] With high prevalence of opioid use in the elderly, the failure to recognize the history of chronic opioid use and presence of chronic pain can result in undertreatment of pain in the perioperative period. The elderly also responds differently to therapies, usually with less efficacy and more severe adverse reactions.

The functional status of elderly patients and their ability to perform activities of daily living must be evaluated to determine their degree of independence and overall quality

Table 4
Assessment scales for older persons with persistent pain

Instrument	Description	Items	Abstract Thinking	Comments
Numerical rating scale (NRS)	Numerical rating via an 11-point scale, ranging from 0 (no pain) to 10 (worst pain)	Numbers: ranging from 0 (no pain) to 10 (worst pain)	Moderate	Appropriate first-line pain-rating instrument in cognitively intact older persons Moderate abstract thinking
Visual analog scale (VAS)	Continuous rating via designating a position along a line	Position designated along line between 2 end points (no pain, worst possible pain)	Significant	Ideal for research given wide range of applicable statistical methods Use of pencil/paper or device to designate position is cumbersome for frail older persons Significant abstract thinking
Verbal rating scale (VRS) or verbal descriptor scale (VDS)	Verbal rating via 4-item categorical scale Instruments up to 7 items available	Descriptions: "none," "mild," "moderate," "severe"	Moderate	Limited number of responses and higher language demand Easy to use in clinical environment but insufficient for research purposes Moderate abstract thinking
Facial pain scale (FPS)	Pictorial rating via 6-item categorical scale 7-, 9-, and 11-item instruments available	Drawings: a series of faces arranged in order of increasing pain expressions	Moderate	Validated in older persons including minority groups Moderate abstract thinking
Pain thermometer	Verbal rating via 6-item categorical scale arranged in vertical order adjacent to image of a thermometer	Descriptions: ranging from "no pain"/white color at base to "pain as bad as could be"/red color at top	Minimal	Validated in older persons with cognitive impairment Minimal abstract thinking

of life.[61] A history of cognitive impairment, delirium, dementia, or falls provides a baseline reference of the patient's cognitive ability and aids the choice of pain assessment tool and multimodal agents to be used for pain management.

Comprehensive education entails reinforcing the importance of adequate pain control to optimize participation in postoperative recovery activities such as incentive spirometry and ambulation and in order to decrease postoperative delirium and functional decline.[62] Realistic expectations need to be set and conveyed that postoperative pain may not be completely abolished but may be minimized through multimodal pain management techniques. The available pain assessment tools need to be introduced preoperatively to ensure that the elderly patient comprehends how to use them.[63]

Treatment options including pharmacologic and nonpharmacologic modalities need to be discussed at the preoperative visit. Misconceptions and fears regarding addiction and tolerance of pain medications, particularly opioids, can interfere with the willingness to take them.[64] Nonpharmacologic treatments including distraction strategies, guided imagery, and mindful breathing should be introduced preoperatively to ensure that they have the physical and mental ability to use them.[65]

Pain control postoperatively requires a fine balance between the adequate treatment of pain and the avoidance of overtreatment with opioids. A dose reduction of 25% to 50% of the adult opioid dose is appropriate to start.[66] The dose is increased by 25% until there is a 50% reduction in pain or the patient reports satisfactory pain relief. If changing opioid agents or routes of administration, the new dose should be calculated based on an equianalgesic table and lowered by 25% to 50% to account for incomplete cross-tolerance. The oral route is preferred over the intravenous route given the latter's increased risk of adverse events such as sedation, respiratory depression, cognitive impairment, and postoperative delirium.[67] Patients on chronic opioids, especially those with opioid tolerance, present a unique subset that may require larger than usual doses of opioids postoperatively; this is especially true for moderately to severely painful surgeries. The challenge then becomes balancing adequate pain control with the required opioid doses, while preventing dangerous side effects of respiratory depression and oversedation related to an overdose.

Multimodal regimens that incorporate nonpharmacologic and nonopioid agents help reduce adverse effects of opioids. Notable nonopioid agents include acetaminophen and nonsteroidal antiinflammatory drugs (NSAIDs). Acetaminophen is well tolerated by the elderly; can be administered orally, rectally, and intravenously; has a favorable safety profile; and has shown that a single dose given preoperatively can reduce early pain and postoperative opioid consumption.[68] NSAIDs are included in the Beers criteria due to the increased risk of gastrointestinal bleed, peptic ulcer disease, and acute kidney injury.[69] However, this pertains to chronic NSAID usage. Administration in the immediate perioperative period has not been associated with bleeding or renal dysfunction, and a single preoperative dose of ketorolac reduces early pain and postoperative opioid consumption.[68] When given preoperatively to patients undergoing total knee arthroplasty, celecoxib decreased opioid consumption, pain scores, and sleep disturbances, leading to shortened recovery time.[70] Similarly, preoperative and postoperative oral celecoxib in a multimodal analgesic strategy can achieve favorable pain relief, reduce opioid consumption, and provide earlier ambulation and improved rehabilitation when compared with patient-controlled analgesia morphine alone, following total hip arthroplasty in elderly patients.[71]

Regional analgesia techniques provide site-specific analgesia with minimal side effects and thus are ideal choices for perioperative pain control in the elderly population. Benefits include postoperative reduction of pain scores and need for analgesic medications (including opioids), earlier ambulation, earlier return of bowel function, prevention of pulmonary complications, improved mental status, decreased postoperative delirium, functional decline, nausea and vomiting, and decreased discharge time.[59] For abdominal surgeries, ilioinguinal-hypogastric, paravertebral, and transversus abdominis plane blocks improve recovery.[72] For orthopedic surgeries, single-shot interscalene, femoral, and popliteal-sciatic blocks provide improved pain control with less bowel and bladder dysfunction compared with opioid-based analgesic techniques.[73] In addition, continuous local anesthetics infusions can provide opioid-sparing pain relief directly to a surgical site for up to 5 days.[74] Of note, although regional techniques provide superior pain relief, it is important to be cognizant of the effects of a dense motor block and altered sensation that may be dangerous for the elderly, especially after ambulatory surgery.[75] Such techniques therefore require careful titration of local anesthetics to avoid impairment of motor function and delays in functional rehabilitation.

Pain Management for Nonsurgical Inpatients and Nursing Home Residents

A study analyzing the prevalence, nature, and severity of pain and its pharmacologic treatment in elderly patients hospitalized in medical wards found that 23.2% patients experienced pain; 73.4% of patients with chronic pain were not treated at the time of admission and at hospital discharge, and 50.5% of patients with chronic pain remained untreated. The investigators believed that undertreatment and poor pain relief reflected an underestimation of the importance of pain in the elderly and/or the potential poor expertise on pain assessment and treatment by the physicians involved.[76] Similarly, a study by Lukas and colleagues performed in nursing home residents found that up to 24% of residents reporting pain did not receive any pain medication and 11% received it only on an as-needed basis (as opposed to regularly scheduled), regardless of pain intensity. Sixty-one percent of nursing home residents also did not receive any nonpharmacologic treatment of their pain.[77]

Recently, guidelines by the Centers of Disease Control and Prevention regarding the prescribing of opioids in non–cancer-related pain is designed to discourage opioid use for routine pain management in those with chronic pain and exclude those who are near the end of life or are on palliative care. The guidelines state that although opioids can reduce pain during short-term use, the review found insufficient evidence to determine whether pain relief is sustained and whether function or quality of life improves with long-term opioid therapy. Although benefits for pain relief, function, and quality of life with long-term opioid use for chronic pain are uncertain, risks associated with long-term opioid use are clear and significant, including potential risks such as opioid use disorder, overdose, myocardial infarction, and motor vehicle injury.[78] However, many geriatric experts consider nursing home residents as palliative patients and are proponents of focusing on quality of life, especially in those with limited life expectancies. They argue that many nursing home residents do not have the life expectancy required to develop tolerance to escalating doses of opioids.[79] Ultimately, initiating opioids and keeping nursing home residents on scheduled opioids is a clinical decision, and benefits need to be weighed against risks in each clinical context.

When evaluating pain in the elderly in nursing homes, it is important to bear in mind that cognitive impairment can lead to memory, language, and speech deficits that could limit clear communication about pain and discomfort.[53] In these cases, observation-based assessments including pain behaviors and collateral information from family or caregivers, over verbal assessments such as the NRS, are preferred to assess and treat pain.[80] Optimal pharmacologic treatment includes the rapid institution of pain treatment because the potential for unrelieved and unrecognized pain is greater in this population who cannot reliably express their discomfort.[53] Geriatric experts recommend the use of a scheduled rather than an as-needed regimen for chronic or predictably recurrent pain. For example, scheduled low-dose, long-acting opioids lessened agitation in patients 85 years and older in nursing homes with advanced dementia.[81] Similar to the treatment of patients with intact cognition, titration of medication to pain level based on verbal, behavioral, and functional responses and frequent reassessment of responses to treatment are important, especially because patients with dementia experience less intense pain, less affective distress, and a blunted autonomic response compared with the cognitively intact patients.[82] Key side effects to consider include sedation, respiratory depression, impairment of cognition and balance, gastrointestinal bleeding, and constipation. Nonpharmacologic approaches such as, physical exercise, cognitive-behavioral therapy, patient pain education, acupuncture, transcutaneous nerve stimulation, chiropractic, heat, cold, massage, relaxation, and distraction techniques are an integral part of pain management.[80] In the cognitively impaired, approaches that do not require significant cognitive ability are preferred. In addition, it is important to appropriately pace the activities with adequate sensory stimulating and calming activities, for inappropriate pacing can lead to increased levels of agitation in patients with dementia.[83]

PAIN MANAGEMENT IN OUTPATIENT SETTINGS

Currently a large proportion of the literature surrounding pain management in the elderly focuses on the perioperative period. As such, the recommendations may overlap somewhat in terms of the treatment of pain for the elderly in the outpatient setting. The treatment of pain in the elderly can be divided into 2 broad categories: nonpharmacologic and pharmacologic management.

Nonpharmacologic treatments include heat and ice, complementary therapies, mental health support, as well as physical activity and therapy.

Heat and ice are commonly used to treat pain in the outpatient setting. Heat is often used for situations with stiffness or poor blood flow. Cold, on the other hand, is used to reduce blood flow, thereby decreasing inflammation, and bruising while numbing the area. Although there are no data specific to the elderly population concerning this modality of treatment, a Cochrane review looking at thermotherapy for the treatment of osteoarthritis found that although cold therapy resulted in decreased swelling and increased range of motion, function, and strength, it did not affect intensity of pain significantly. Heat also did not have significant effects on edema or pain.[84] A randomized controlled trial had similar findings when looking at heat and transcutaneous electrical nerve stimulation (TENS) for the treatment of low back pain, showing that although pain pressure thresholds were improved, there was no reduction in pain scores.

Complementary therapies include neurostimulation, acupuncture, and even massage. Leemans and colleagues showed that neurostimulation was not effective for low back pain.[85] Contrary to those findings, however, Simon and colleagues found TENS was useful not only in older adults aged 57 to 79 years, but younger patients as well for axial back pain.[86] Specifically, there was a reduction in resting pain, movement-related pain, as well as improved function.[86] Acupuncture and massage therapy have shown some benefit for osteoarthritic knee pain, although the studies were not limited to elderly patients.[87,88]

It seems that mental health and psychological support can play a role in reducing chronic pain in the elderly. A review by Lunde and colleagues noted that cognitive behavioral therapy was an effective treatment modality for chronic pain in the elderly

Table 5
Recommended drugs for persistent pain in older adults

Drug	Starting Dose	Comments
Acetaminophen (Tylenol)	325–500 mg every 4 h or 500–1000 mg every 6 h Maximum dose usually 4 g daily.	Reduce maximum dose by 50% to 75% in patients with hepatic insufficiency or history of alcohol abuse
NSAIDs		
Celecoxib (Celebrex)	100 mg daily	Higher doses associated with higher incidence of gastrointestinal, cardiovascular side effects. Patients with indications for cardioprotection require aspirin supplement; therefore, older individuals will still require concurrent gastroprotection.
Naproxen sodium	220 mg twice daily	Several studies implicate this agent as possessing less cardiovascular toxicity.
Ibuprofen	200 mg 3 times a day	Food and Drug Administration indicates concurrent use with aspirin inhibits aspirin's antiplatelet effect, but the true clinical import of this remains to be elucidated, and it remains unclear whether this is unique to ibuprofen or true with other NSAIDs.
Diclofenac sodium	50 mg twice daily or 75 mg extended release daily	Owing to its relative cyclooxygenase-2 inhibitor selectivity, this agent may be associated with higher cardiovascular risk compared with other traditional NSAIDs.
Opioids		
Hydrocodone	2.5–5 mg every 4–6 h	Useful for acute recurrent, episodic, or breakthrough pain; daily dose limited by fixed-dose combinations with acetaminophen or NSAIDs. Prescribers need to consider the amount of nonopioid agent in each of these preparations (they are not all the same) and other acetaminophen or NSAID-containing preparations the patient is taking, including over-the-counter medications.
Oxycodone	2.5–5 mg every 4–6 h	Useful for acute recurrent, episodic, or breakthrough pain; daily immediate-release dose limited by fixed-dose combinations with acetaminophen or NSAIDs. Immediate-release oxycodone is available without added coanalgesics. Prescribers should specify which oxycodone preparation they want for their patient to avoid confusion or coanalgesic toxicity.

Drug	Dose	Comments
Oxycontin	10 mg every 12 h	Usually started after initial dose determined by effects of immediate release opioid or as an alternative to a different long-acting opioid because of indications for opioid rotation. Although intended for 12-h dosing, some patients only get 8 h of effective analgesia, whereas some frail older patients get 12–24 h of relief
Morphine immediate release	2.5–10 mg every 4 h	Available in tablet form and as concentrated oral solution, which is most used for episodic or breakthrough pain and for patients unable to swallow tablets.
Morphine sustained release	15 mg every 8–24 h	Usually started after initial dose determined by effects of immediate release opioid or as an alternative to a different long-acting opioid due to indications for opioid rotation. Toxic metabolites of morphine may limit usefulness in patients with renal insufficiency or when high-dose therapy is required. Continuous-release formulations may require more frequent dosing if end-of-dose failure occurs regularly. Significant interactions with food and alcohol toxicity.
Hydromorphone	1–2 mg every 3 h	For breakthrough pain or for around-the-clock dosing
Antidepressants		
Amitriptyline, nortriptyline	10 mg at bedtime	Significant risk of adverse effects in older patients. Anticholinergic effects (visual, urinary, gastrointestinal); cardiovascular effects (orthostasis, atrioventricular blockade). Older persons rarely tolerate doses >75–100 mg/d.
Duloxetine	20 mg daily	Monitor blood pressure, dizziness, cognitive effects, and memory. Has multiple drug–drug interactions.
Anticonvulsants		
Carbamazepine	100 mg daily	Monitor hepatic transaminases (aspartate transaminase, alanine transaminase), complete blood count, creatinine, blood urea nitrogen, electrolytes, serum carbamazepine levels. Multiple drug–drug interactions.
Gabapentin	100 mg at bedtime	Monitor sedation, ataxia, edema
Pregabalin	50 mg at bedtime	Monitor sedation, ataxia, edema

(continued on next page)

Table 5
(continued)

Drug	Starting Dose	Comments
Muscle Relaxants		
Baclofen	5 mg up to 3 times daily	Monitor muscle weakness, urinary function, cognitive effects, sedation. Avoid abrupt discontinuation because of central nervous system irritability. Older persons rarely tolerate doses >30–40 mg/d.
Tizanidine	2 mg up to 3 times daily	Monitor muscle weakness, urinary function, cognitive effects, sedation, orthostasis. Potential for many drug–drug interactions.
Clonazepam	0.25–0.5 mg at bedtime	Monitor sedation, memory, complete blood count.
Mixed Mechanism		
Tramadol	12.5–25 mg every 4–6 h	Mixed opioid and norepinephrine or serotonin reuptake inhibitor mechanisms of action. Monitor for opioid side effects, including drowsiness, constipation, and nausea. Risk of seizures if used in high doses or in predisposed patients. May precipitate serotonin syndrome if used with selective serotonin reuptake inhibitors.
Tapentadol	50 mg every 4–6 h	Clinical trials of tapentadol suggest lower incidence of gastrointestinal adverse events than comparator opioids.

with regard to self-reported pain experience.[89] In addition, a mind-body program has been shown to improve pain, physical, and psychological function in older adults with low back pain.[90]

Physical activity and therapy seem to be beneficial for older adults with knee osteoarthritis, in reducing pain and improving function.[91,92] However, when looking at physical therapy in patients with hip osteoarthritis, one study showed there was no greater improvement in pain or function compared with the sham group.[93]

When considering pharmacologic management of elderly patients, it is important to consider the physiologic changes with aging that affect the pharmacokinetics and pharmacodynamics of medications. The lean mass and total body water content are decreased, whereas body fat increases, affecting volume of distribution, plasma concentration, and elimination of drugs. In addition, bones and viscera shrink and basal metabolic rate decreases, resulting in profound modifications in dosage and drug metabolism of analgesic drugs. These changes are difficult to quantify and vary from person to person.[55] In terms of dosing, the American Geriatrics Society has developed guidelines to help with the pharmacologic management of pain in the elderly population. A particularly useful tool is a table that was developed with recommended drugs to use for pain in older adults, which was abbreviated and reproduced in **Table 5**.[58]

Given the potential for increased risk of adverse events from medications, there exists a unique and important role for interventional therapies in the elderly population for the management of chronic pain. In general, interventional modalities are most easily assessed when considering pathologies that involve discrete anatomic targets, for example, when considering treatment of osteoarthritic pain, chronic back pain, or neuropathic pain. Pharmacologic agents are deposited in discrete aliquots to target specific generators of pain and reduce or delay systemic absorption. One should note that interventions such as epidural steroid injections, intraarticular joint injections, and advanced therapies (spinal cord stimulation and intrathecal drug delivery) although proved to be effective in the general population (for all ages) for the treatment of chronic pain, their efficacy has not been specifically studied in the elderly. When offering steroid injections to the elderly, it is imperative to be cognizant of side effects from multiple steroid doses specifically in the elderly patient. Lowest effective dose of steroid and use of nonparticulate steroids seem to balance efficacy with risk.

SUMMARY

Pain assessment and treatment remains challenging in the elderly population. Elderly patients underreport pain, assuming it to be a normal part of aging and physicians undertreat pain. Nonpharmacologic and interventional options, besides medications, need to be studied further in the elderly population.

CLINICS CARE POINTS

- Pain perception changes with aging.
- Increased pain threshold that accompanies aging may imply that more significant levels of underlying pathologic disorder may be present in older adults who endorse pain.
- Elderly patients likely have more than one cause contributing to their chronic pain and therefore treatment of one causative factor will not necessarily address all aspects of a patient's experience of chronic pain.

- Older adults with cognitive impairment may demonstrate a variety of behaviors to communicate pain, including facial expressions, verbalization, body movements, and changes in interactions with other people and their environment.
- Management of perioperative pain in the elderly patients should focus on history of chronic painful conditions, physical examination, comprehensive education, and utilization of opioid-sparing and multimodal pain management techniques.

FUNDING SOURCES

none.

CONFLICTS OF INTEREST

no conflicts for any of the authors.

FINANCIAL DISCLOSURES

none.

AUTHORS' STATEMENT

The manuscript has been read and approved by all the authors, the requirements for authorship have been met, and each author believes that the manuscript represents honest work.

REFERENCES

1. Roberts A.W., Ogunwole S.U., Blakeslee L., Rabe M.A., The Population 65 Years and Older in the United States. United States Census Bureau. 2018. Available at: https://www.census.gov/library/publications/2018/acs/acs-38.html.
2. Molton IR, Terrill AL. Overview of persistent pain in older adults. Am Psychol 2014;69(2):197.
3. Cavalieri TA. Pain management in the elderly. J Osteopath Med 2002;102(9): 481–5.
4. Mercadante S, Arcuri E. Pharmacological management of cancer pain in the elderly. Drugs & aging 2007;24(9):761–76.
5. Gianni W, Madaio RA, Di Cioccio L, et al. Prevalence of pain in elderly hospitalized patients. Arch Gerontol Geriatr 2010;51(3):273–6.
6. American Geriatrics Society Recommends Opioids as Second-Line Therapy for Chronic Pain, Instead of NSAIDs. Top Pain Manag 2009;25(1):9–10.
7. Jakobsson U, Klevsgård R, Westergren A, et al. Old people in pain: a comparative study. J Pain Symptom Manag 2003;26(1):625–36.
8. Brattberg G, Parker MG, Thorslund M. A longitudinal study of pain: reported pain from middle age to old age. Clin J Pain 1997;13(2):144–9.
9. Helme RD, Gibson SJ. The epidemiology of pain in elderly people. Clin Geriatr Med 2001;17(3):417–31.
10. Patel KV, Guralnik JM, Dansie EJ, et al. Prevalence and impact of pain among older adults in the United States: findings from the 2011 National Health and Aging Trends Study. Pain® 2013;154(12):2649–57.
11. Smith AK, Cenzer IS, Knight SJ, et al. The epidemiology of pain during the last 2 years of life. Annals of internal medicine 2010;153(9):563–9.

12. Abdulla A, Adams N, Bone M, et al. Guidance on the management of pain in older people. Age Ageing 2013;42:i1–57.
13. Malec M, Shega JW. Pain management in the elderly. Medical Clinics 2015;99(2): 337–50.
14. Maxwell CJ, Dalby DM, Slater M, et al. The prevalence and management of current daily pain among older home care clients. Pain 2008;138(1):208–16.
15. Shega JW, Tiedt AD, Grant K, et al. Pain measurement in the National Social Life, Health, and Aging Project: presence, intensity, and location. J Gerontol B Psychol Sci Soc Sci 2014;69(Suppl_2):S191–7.
16. Lowsky DJ, Olshansky SJ, Bhattacharya J, et al. Heterogeneity in healthy aging. Journals of Gerontology Series A: Biomedical Sciences and Medical Sciences 2014;69(6):640–9.
17. Fine PG. Chronic pain management in older adults: special considerations. J Pain Symptom Manag 2009;38(2):S4–14.
18. Karp JF, Shega JW, Morone NE, et al. Advances in understanding the mechanisms and management of persistent pain in older adults. British journal of anaesthesia 2008;101(1):111–20.
19. Gibson S. Pain and aging: The pain experience over the adult life span. Progress in Pain Research and Management 2003;24:767–90.
20. Cole LJ, Farrell MJ, Gibson SJ, et al. Age-related differences in pain sensitivity and regional brain activity evoked by noxious pressure. Neurobiol Aging 2010; 31(3):494–503.
21. Riley JL III, Cruz-Almeida Y, Glover TL, et al. Age and race effects on pain sensitivity and modulation among middle-aged and older adults. J Pain 2014;15(3): 272–82.
22. Hilton D, Iman N, Burke G, et al. Absence of abdominal pain in older persons with endoscopic ulcers: a prospective study. Am J Gastroenterol 2001;96(2):380–4.
23. Mehta RH, Rathore SS, Radford MJ, et al. Acute myocardial infarction in the elderly: differences by age. J Am Coll Cardiol 2001;38(3):736–41.
24. Bicket MC, Mao J. Chronic pain in older adults. Anesthesiol Clin 2015;33(3): 577–90.
25. Dimitroulas T, Duarte RV, Behura A, et al. Neuropathic pain in osteoarthritis: a review of pathophysiological mechanisms and implications for treatment. Semin Arthritis Rheum 2014;44(2):145–54.
26. Williams C., and Jimenez S.A., "Molecular biology of heritable cartilage disorders." *Osteoarthritic disorders. Rosemont: American Academy of Orthopaedic Surgeons* ,1995, 35-50.
27. Sharma L, Kapoor D, Issa S. Epidemiology of osteoarthritis: an update. Curr Opin Rheumatol 2006;18(2):147–56.
28. Aletaha D, Funovits J, Smolen JS. Physical disability in rheumatoid arthritis is associated with cartilage damage rather than bone destruction. Ann Rheum Dis 2011;70(5):733–9.
29. Aletaha D, Smolen JS. Diagnosis and management of rheumatoid arthritis: a review. JAMA 2018;320(13):1360–72.
30. Jansson K-Å, Blomqvist P, Granath F, et al. Spinal stenosis surgery in Sweden 1987–1999. Eur Spine J 2003;12(5):535–41.
31. Melancia JL, Francisco AF, Antunes JL. Spinal stenosis. Handb Clin Neurol 2014; 119:541–9.
32. Baker AD. Abnormal magnetic-resonance scans of the lumbar spine in asymptomatic subjects. A prospective investigation, . Classic papers in orthopaedics. Springer; 2014. p. 245–7.

33. Veves A, Backonja M, Malik RA. Painful diabetic neuropathy: epidemiology, natural history, early diagnosis, and treatment options. Pain Med 2008;9(6):660–74.

34. Pickering G. Antiepileptics for post-herpetic neuralgia in the elderly: current and future prospects. Drugs & aging 2014;31(9):653–60.

35. Stewart KJ, Hiatt WR, Regensteiner JG, et al. Exercise training for claudication. N Engl J Med 2002;347(24):1941–51.

36. Selvin E, Erlinger TP. Prevalence of and risk factors for peripheral arterial disease in the United States: results from the National Health and Nutrition Examination Survey, 1999–2000. Circulation 2004;110(6):738–43.

37. De Toledo IP, Réus JC, Fernandes M, et al. Prevalence of trigeminal neuralgia: A systematic review. The Journal of the American Dental Association 2016;147(7): 570–6. e2.

38. Araya EI, Claudino RF, Piovesan EJ, et al. Trigeminal neuralgia: basic and clinical aspects. Curr Neuropharmacol 2020;18(2):109–19.

39. Naess H, Lunde L, Brogger J. The effects of fatigue, pain, and depression on quality of life in ischemic stroke patients: the Bergen Stroke Study. Vasc Health Risk Manag 2012;8:407.

40. Klit H, Finnerup NB, Andersen G, et al. Central poststroke pain: a population-based study. PAIN® 2011;152(4):818–24.

41. Sommerfeld D, Welmer AK. Pain following stroke, initially and at 3 and 18 months after stroke, and its association with other disabilities. Eur J Neurol 2012;19(10): 1325–30.

42. Van den Beuken-van Everdingen M, De Rijke J, Kessels A, et al. Prevalence of pain in patients with cancer: a systematic review of the past 40 years. Ann Oncol 2007;18(9):1437–49.

43. Hackett J, Godfrey M, Bennett MI. Patient and caregiver perspectives on managing pain in advanced cancer: a qualitative longitudinal study. Palliative medicine 2016;30(8):711–9.

44. Portenoy RK. Treatment of cancer pain. Lancet 2011;377(9784):2236–47.

45. Deyo RA, Mirza SK, Martin BI. Back pain prevalence and visit rates: estimates from US national surveys, 2002. Spine 2006;31(23):2724–7.

46. Schug S.A. and Bruce J., Risk stratification for the development of chronic post-surgical pain, *Pain Rep*, 2 (6), 2017, e627.

47. Katz J, Seltzer Ze. Transition from acute to chronic postsurgical pain: risk factors and protective factors. Expert Rev Neurother 2009;9(5):723–44.

48. VanDenKerkhof EG, Peters ML, Bruce J. Chronic pain after surgery: time for standardization? A framework to establish core risk factor and outcome domains for epidemiological studies. Clin J Pain 2013;29(1):2–8.

49. Malec M, Shega JW. Pain Management in the Elderly. Med Clin 2015;99(2): 337–50.

50. Weiner DK, Karp JF, Bernstein CD, et al. Pain medicine in older adults: how should it differ? Comprehensive treatment of chronic pain by medical, interventional, and Integrative approaches. Springer; 2013. p. 977–1002.

51. Raja SN, Sommer CL. Pain 2014 Refresher Courses: 15th World Congress on pain. In: Comprehensive Treatment of Chronic Pain by Medical, Interventional, and Integrative Approaches. Lippincott Williams & Wilkins; 2015.

52. Hadjistavropoulos T, Herr K, Turk DC, et al. An interdisciplinary expert consensus statement on assessment of pain in older persons. Pain 2014 Refresher Courses: 15th World Congress on Pain 2007;23:S1–43.

53. Buffum MD, Hutt E, Chang VT, et al. Cognitive impairment and pain management: review of issues and challenges. Journal of rehabilitation research and development 2007;44(2):315.
54. Gallasch CH, Alexandre NMC. The measurement of musculoskeletal pain intensity: a comparison of four methods. Revista Gaúcha de Enfermagem. 2007; 28(2):260.
55. Jones MR, Ehrhardt KP, Ripoll JG, et al. Pain in the Elderly. Curr Pain Headache Rep 2016;20(4):23.
56. Herr KA, Spratt K, Mobily PR, et al. Pain intensity assessment in older adults: use of experimental pain to compare psychometric properties and usability of selected pain scales with younger adults. Clin J Pain 2004;20(4):207–19.
57. Society AG. Panel on Persistent Pain in Older Persons. The management of persistent pain in older adults. J Am Geriatr Soc 2002;50(6):205–24.
58. Persons O. Pharmacological management of persistent pain in older persons. J Am Geriatr Soc 2009;57(8):1331–46.
59. Shellito AD, Dworsky JQ, Kirkland PJ, et al. Perioperative pain management issues unique to older adults undergoing surgery: A narrative review. Annals of Surgery Open 2021;2(3):e072.
60. Campbell CI, Weisner C, LeResche L, et al. Age and gender trends in long-term opioid analgesic use for noncancer pain. American journal of public health 2010; 100(12):2541–7.
61. Herr K. Pain Assessment in Cognitively Impaired Older Adults: New strategies and careful observation help pinpoint unspoken pain. AJN The American Journal of Nursing 2002;102(12):65–7.
62. McGory ML, Kao KK, Shekelle PG, et al. Developing quality indicators for elderly surgical patients. Annals of surgery 2009;250(2):338–47.
63. Ware LJ, Epps CD, Herr K, et al. Evaluation of the revised faces pain scale, verbal descriptor scale, numeric rating scale, and Iowa pain thermometer in older minority adults. Pain Manag Nurs 2006;7(3):117–25.
64. Ardery G, Herr KA, Titler MG, et al. Assessing and managing acute pain in older adults: a research base to guide practice. Medsurg Nurs 2003;12(1):7.
65. Tick H, Nielsen A, Pelletier KR, et al. Evidence-based nonpharmacologic strategies for comprehensive pain care: the consortium pain task force white paper. Explore 2018;14(3):177–211.
66. Naples JG, Gellad WF, Hanlon JT. The role of opioid analgesics in geriatric pain management. Clin Geriatr Med 2016;32(4):725–35.
67. McKeown JL. Pain management issues for the geriatric surgical patient. Anesthesiol Clin 2015;33(3):563–76.
68. De Oliveira GS Jr, Castro-Alves LJ, McCarthy RJ. Single-dose systemic acetaminophen to prevent postoperative pain: a meta-analysis of randomized controlled trials. Clin J Pain 2015;31(1):86–93.
69. White PF, Tang J, Wender RH, et al. The Effects of Oral Ibuprofen and Celecoxib in Preventing Pain, Improving Recovery Outcomes and Patient Satisfaction After Ambulatory Surgery. Surv Anesthesiol 2012;56(1):1.
70. Ji Z, Bao N, Zhao J, et al. Effect of preoperative cyclooxygenase-2 inhibitor for postoperative pain in patients after total knee arthroplasty: a meta-analysis. Zhongguo gu Shang= China Journal of Orthopaedics and Traumatology 2015; 28(9):838–45.
71. Chen J, Zhu W, Zhang Z, et al. Efficacy of celecoxib for acute pain management following total hip arthroplasty in elderly patients: A prospective, randomized, placebo-control trial. Exp Ther Med 2015;10(2):737–42.

72. Song D, Greilich NB, White PF, et al. Recovery profiles and costs of anesthesia for outpatient unilateral inguinal herniorrhaphy. Anesth Analg 2000;91(4):876–81.
73. Amin NH, West JA, Farmer T, et al. Nerve blocks in the geriatric patient with hip fracture: A review of the current literature and relevant neuroanatomy. Geriatr Orthop Surg Rehabil 2017;8(4):268–75.
74. Liang S.S., Ying A.J., Affan E.T., et al., Continuous local anaesthetic wound infusion for postoperative pain after midline laparotomy for colorectal resection in adults, Cochrane Database Syst Rev, 10 (10), 2019, CD012310.
75. Cao X, Elvir-Lazo OL, White PF, et al. An update on pain management for elderly patients undergoing ambulatory surgery. Current Opinion in Anesthesiology 2016;29(6):674–82.
76. Corsi N, Roberto A, Cortesi L, et al. Prevalence, characteristics and treatment of chronic pain in elderly patients hospitalized in internal medicine wards. Eur J Intern Med 2018;55:35–9.
77. Lukas A, Mayer B, Fialová D, et al. Pain characteristics and pain control in European nursing homes: cross-sectional and longitudinal results from the Services and Health for Elderly in Long TERm care (SHELTER) study. J Am Med Dir Assoc 2013;14(6):421–8.
78. Dowell D, Haegerich TM, Chou R. CDC guideline for prescribing opioids for chronic pain—United States, 2016. JAMA 2016;315(15):1624–45.
79. Sanford AM. Pain management in the elderly. J Am Med Dir Assoc 2016;17(8): 678–9.
80. Stolee P, Hillier LM, Esbaugh J, et al. Instruments for the assessment of pain in older persons with cognitive impairment. J Am Geriatr Soc 2005;53(2):319–26.
81. Manfredi PL, Breuer B, Wallenstein S, et al. Opioid treatment for agitation in patients with advanced dementia. Int J Geriatr Psychiatr 2003;18(8):700–5.
82. Rainero I, Vighetti S, Bergamasco B, et al. Autonomic responses and pain perception in Alzheimer's disease. Eur J Pain 2000;4(3):267–74.
83. Kovach CR, Wells T. Pacing of activity as a predictor of agitation for persons with dementia in acute care. NJ: SLACK Incorporated Thorofare; 2002. p. 28–35.
84. Brosseau L., Yonge K., Welch V., et al., Thermotherapy for treatment of osteoarthritis, Cochrane Database Syst Rev, 2003 (4), 2003, CD004522.
85. Leemans L, Elma Ö, Nijs J, et al. Transcutaneous electrical nerve stimulation and heat to reduce pain in a chronic low back pain population: a randomized controlled clinical trial. Braz J Phys Ther 2021;25(1):86–96.
86. Simon CB, Riley JL III, Fillingim RB, et al. Age group comparisons of TENS response among individuals with chronic axial low back pain. J Pain 2015; 16(12):1268–79.
87. Manheimer E, Linde K, Lao L, et al. Meta-analysis: acupuncture for osteoarthritis of the knee. Annals of internal medicine 2007;146(12):868–77.
88. Perlman AI, Sabina A, Williams A-L, et al. Massage therapy for osteoarthritis of the knee: a randomized controlled trial. Arch Intern Med 2006;166(22):2533–8.
89. Lunde L-H, Nordhus IH, Pallesen S. The effectiveness of cognitive and behavioural treatment of chronic pain in the elderly: a quantitative review. J Clin Psychol Med Settings 2009;16(3):254–62.
90. Morone NE, Greco CM, Moore CG, et al. A mind-body program for older adults with chronic low back pain: a randomized clinical trial. JAMA Intern Med 2016; 176(3):329–37.
91. Deyle GD, Henderson NE, Matekel RL, et al. Effectiveness of manual physical therapy and exercise in osteoarthritis of the knee: a randomized, controlled trial. Annals of Internal Medicine 2000;132(3):173–81.

92. Focht BC. Effectiveness of exercise interventions in reducing pain symptoms among older adults with knee osteoarthritis: a review. J Aging Phys Activ 2006; 14(2):212–35.
93. Bennell KL, Egerton T, Martin J, et al. Effect of physical therapy on pain and function in patients with hip osteoarthritis: a randomized clinical trial. JAMA 2014; 311(19):1987–97.

Printed and bound by CPI Group (UK) Ltd, Croydon, CR0 4YY

08/05/2025

01864749-0009